T0337879

THE SMILE GAP

MCGILL-QUEEN'S/ASSOCIATED MEDICAL SERVICES STUDIES IN THE HISTORY OF MEDICINE, HEALTH, AND SOCIETY
SERIES EDITORS: J.T.H. CONNOR AND ERIKA DYCK

This series presents books in the history of medicine, health studies, and social policy, exploring interactions between the institutions, ideas, and practices of medicine and those of society as a whole. To begin to understand these complex relationships and their history is a vital step to ensuring the protection of a fundamental human right: the right to health. Volumes in this series have received financial support to assist publication from Associated Medical Services, Inc. (AMS), a Canadian charitable organization with an impressive history as a catalyst for change in Canadian healthcare. For eighty years, AMS has had a profound impact through its support of the history of medicine and the education of healthcare professionals, and by making strategic investments to address critical issues in our healthcare system. AMS has funded eight chairs in the history of medicine across Canada, is a primary sponsor of many of the country's history of medicine and nursing organizations, and offers fellowships and grants through the AMS History of Medicine and Healthcare Program (www.amshealthcare.ca).

1 Home Medicine
The Newfoundland Experience
John K. Crellin
2 A Long Way from Home
The Tuberculosis Epidemic among the Inuit
Pat Sandiford Grygier
3 Labrador Odyssey
The Journal and Photographs of Eliot Curwen on the Second Voyage of Wilfred Grenfell, 1893
Ronald Rompkey
4 Architecture in the Family Way
Doctors, Houses, and Women, 1870–1900
Annmarie Adams
5 Local Hospitals in Ancien Régime France
Rationalization, Resistance, Renewal, 1530–1789
Daniel Hickey
6 Foisted upon the Government?
State Responsibilities, Family Obligations, and the Care of the Dependent Aged in Nineteenth-Century Ontario
Edgar-André Montigny
7 A Young Man's Benefit
The Independent Order of Odd Fellows and Sickness Insurance in the United States and Canada, 1860–1929
George Emery and J.C. Herbert Emery
8 The Weariness, the Fever, and the Fret
The Campaign against Tuberculosis in Canada, 1900–1950
Katherine McCuaig
9 The War Diary of Clare Gass, 1915–1918
Edited by Susan Mann
10 Committed to the State Asylum
Insanity and Society in Nineteenth-Century Quebec and Ontario
James E. Moran
11 Jessie Luther at the Grenfell Mission
Edited by Ronald Rompkey
12 Negotiating Disease
Power and Cancer Care, 1900–1950
Barbara Clow
13 For Patients of Moderate Means
A Social History of the Voluntary Public General Hospital in Canada, 1890–1950
David Gagan and Rosemary Gagan
14 Into the House of Old
A History of Residential Care in British Columbia
Megan J. Davies
15 St Mary's
The History of a London Teaching Hospital
E.A. Heaman

16 Women, Health, and Nation
Canada and the United States since 1945
Edited by Georgina Feldberg, Molly Ladd-Taylor, Alison Li, and Kathryn McPherson
17 The Labrador Memoir of Dr Henry Paddon, 1912–1938
Edited by Ronald Rompkey
18 J.B. Collip and the Development of Medical Research in Canada
Extracts and Enterprise
Alison Li
19 The Ontario Cancer Institute
Successes and Reverses at Sherbourne Street
E.A. McCulloch
20 Island Doctor
John Mackieson and Medicine in Nineteenth-Century Prince Edward Island
David A.E. Shephard
21 The Struggle to Serve
A History of the Moncton Hospital, 1895 to 1953
W.G. Godfrey
22 An Element of Hope
Radium and the Response to Cancer in Canada, 1900–1940
Charles Hayter
23 Labour in the Laboratory
Medical Laboratory Workers in the Maritimes, 1900–1950
Peter L. Twohig
24 Rockefeller Foundation Funding and Medical Education in Toronto, Montreal, and Halifax
Marianne P. Fedunkiw
25 Push!
The Struggle for Midwifery in Ontario
Ivy Lynn Bourgeault
26 Mental Health and Canadian Society
Historical Perspectives
Edited by James Moran and David Wright
27 SARS in Context
Memory, History, and Policy
Edited by Jacalyn Duffin and Arthur Sweetman
28 Lyndhurst
Canada's First Rehabilitation Centre for People with Spinal Cord Injuries, 1945–1998
Geoffrey Reaume
29 J. Wendell Macleod
Saskatchewan's "Red Dean"
Louis Horlick
30 Who Killed the Queen?
The Story of a Community Hospital and How to Fix Public Health Care
Holly Dressel
31 Healing the World's Children
Interdisciplinary Perspectives on Health in the Twentieth Century
Edited by Cynthia Comacchio, Janet Golden, and George Weisz
32 A Surgeon in the Army of the Potomac
Francis M. Wafer
Edited by Cheryl A. Wells
33 A Sadly Troubled History
The Meanings of Suicide in the Modern Age
John Weaver
34 SARS Unmasked
Risk Communication of Pandemics and Influenza in Canada
Michael G. Tyshenko with assistance from Cathy Patterson
35 Tuberculosis Then and Now
Perspectives on the History of an Infectious Disease
Edited by Flurin Condrau and Michael Worboys
36 Caregiving on the Periphery
Historical Perspectives on Nursing and Midwifery in Canada
Edited by Myra Rutherdale
37 Infection of the Innocents
Wet Nurses, Infants, and Syphilis in France, 1780–1900
Joan Sherwood
38 The Fluorspar Mines of Newfoundland
Their History and the Epidemic of Radiation Lung Cancer
John Martin

39 Small Matters
Canadian Children in Sickness and Health, 1900–1940
Mona Gleason

40 Sorrows of a Century
Interpreting Suicide in New Zealand, 1900–2000
John C. Weaver

41 The Black Doctors of Colonial Lima
Science, Race, and Writing in Colonial and Early Republican Peru
José R. Jouve Martín

42 Bodily Subjects
Essays on Gender and Health, 1800–2000
Edited by Tracy Penny Light, Barbara Brookes, and Wendy Mitchinson

43 Expelling the Plague
The Health Office and the Implementation of Quarantine in Dubrovnik, 1377–1533
Zlata Blažina Tomić and Vesna Blažina

44 Telling the Flesh
Life Writing, Citizenship and the Body in the Letters to Samuel Auguste Tissot
Sonja Boon

45 Mobilizing Mercy
A History of the Canadian Red Cross
Sarah Glassford

46 The Invisible Injured
Psychological Trauma in the Canadian Military from the First World War to Afghanistan
Adam Montgomery

47 Carving a Niche
The Medical Profession in Mexico, 1800–1870
Luz María Hernández Sáenz

48 Psychedelic Prophets
The Letters of Aldous Huxley and Humphry Osmond
Edited by Cynthia Carson Bisbee, Paul Bisbee, Erika Dyck, Patrick Farrell, James Sexton, and James W. Spisak

49 The Grenfell Medical Mission and American Support in Newfoundland and Labrador, 1890s–1940s
Edited by Jennifer J. Connor and Katherine Side

50 Broken
Institutions, Families, and the Construction of Intellectual Disability
Madeline C. Burghardt

51 Strange Trips
Science, Culture, and the Regulation of Drugs
Lucas Richert

52 A New Field in Mind
A History of Interdisciplinarity in the Early Brain Sciences
Frank W. Stahnisch

53 An Ambulance on Safari
The ANC and the Making of a Health Department in Exile
Melissa Diane Armstrong

54 Challenging Choices
Canada's Population Control in the 1970s
Erika Dyck and Maureen Lux

55 Foreign Practices
Immigrant Doctors and the History of Canadian Medicare
Sasha Mullally and David Wright

56 Ethnopsychiatry
Henri F. Ellenberger
Edited by Emmanuel Delille
Translated by Jonathan Kaplansky

57 In the Public Good
Eugenics and Law in Ontario
C. Elizabeth Koester

58 Transforming Medical Education
Historical Case Studies of Teaching, Learning, and Belonging in Medicine
Edited by Delia Gavrus and Susan Lamb

59 Patterns of Plague
Changing Ideas about Plague in England and France, 1348–1750
Lori Jones

60 The Smile Gap
A History of Oral Health and Social Inequality
Catherine Carstairs

THE SMILE GAP

A History of Oral Health and Social Inequality

Catherine Carstairs

McGill-Queen's University Press
Montreal & Kingston • London • Chicago

ISBN 978-0-2280-1062-3 (cloth)
ISBN 978-0-2280-1063-0 (paper)
ISBN 978-0-2280-1258-0 (ePDF)
ISBN 978-0-2280-1259-7 (ePUB)

Legal deposit second quarter 2022
Bibliothèque nationale du Québec

Printed in Canada on acid-free paper that is 100% ancient forest free (100% post-consumer recycled), processed chlorine free

This book has been published with the help of a grant from the Canadian Federation for the Humanities and Social Sciences, through the Awards to Scholarly Publications Program, using funds provided by the Social Sciences and Humanities Research Council of Canada.

Funded by the Government of Canada | Financé par le gouvernement du Canada

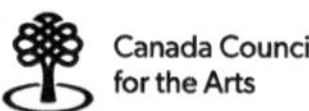

Canada Council for the Arts | Conseil des arts du Canada

We acknowledge the support of the Canada Council for the Arts.

Nous remercions le Conseil des arts du Canada de son soutien.

Library and Archives Canada Cataloguing in Publication

Title: The smile gap : oral health and social inequality / Catherine Carstairs.

Names: Carstairs, Catherine, 1969- author.

Series: McGill-Queen's/Associated Medical Services studies in the history of medicine, health, and society ; 60.

Description: Series statement: McGill-Queen's/Associated Medical Services studies in the history of medicine, health, and society ; 60 | Includes bibliographical references and index.

Identifiers: Canadiana (print) 20220131406 | Canadiana (ebook) 20220131457 | ISBN 9780228010630 (paper) | ISBN 9780228010623 (cloth) | ISBN 9780228012580 (ePDF) | ISBN 9780228012597 (ePUB)

Subjects: LCSH: Dental care – Canada – History. | LCSH: Mouth – Care and hygiene – Canada – History.

Classification: LCC RK52.4.C3 C37 2022 | DDC 362.1976/00971 – dc23

This book was designed and typeset by Peggy & Co. Design in 10.5/13 Sabon.

Contents

Figures

Acknowledgments

This book has been both a very long time and a very short time in the making. I first became interested in the history of oral health when I was studying the history of health food, health-food stores, and natural-health products and realized that many anti-fluoridation campaigns after the Second World War were run out of health-food stores. My work on water fluoridation got me reading the *Journal of the Canadian Dental Association*, and I began to see that there was a much broader story to tell about the history of oral health in Canada. In the meantime, I co-wrote *Be Wise! Be Healthy! Morality, Citizenship and Canadian Public Health Campaigns* (Vancouver: UBC Press, 2018) with two of my former graduate students, Bethany Philpott and Sara Wilmshurst. The subject of our study, the Health League of Canada, was one of the major groups lobbying in favour of fluoridating water after the war. The group started by fighting against sexually transmitted infections (or venereal disease [VD], as it was called at the time) and moved into promoting childhood immunization and a range of other public-health measures. It was a delight to work with people who were as excited about the topic as I was. But as a result, I set aside for a number of years the book you are reading now. My vision of the current project changed substantially over time – I intended initially to focus on the history of the dental professions and state provision of dental care, but my attention shifted to patients' experience, and the manuscript evolved into a more cultural and social history.

The project sputtered along until I received a year's administrative leave from my work at the University of Guelph in 2019. The university has been a collegial and supportive place to work, and I am very grateful for the research, teaching, and administrative opportunities I've had there. My profound thanks as well to my colleagues in the Department of History – they made my being chair a relatively easy task – which left me with the energy to complete most of this manuscript during my administrative leave. In my opinion, being a professor is one of the very best jobs in the world, and I am continually awed at my good luck at being able to do work that I love and that feels meaningful. In the case of this book, I am particularly thankful to the library staff at the University of Guelph, who have tolerated my incessant requests for interlibrary loans with humour and helpfulness, as well as some bewilderment, especially when they received requests for books on sexually transmitted infections and obscure dental journals in the same week. Helen He, Maria Zych, and other staff members at the University of Toronto Dental Library were also incredibly helpful – they tolerated my endless digging through their stacks, my hogging of the photocopy room when it still existed, and my non-stop requests for interlibrary loans.

Many research assistants helped me along the way, including some of the first students I worked with at the University of Guelph: Rachel Elder (now a postdoctoral fellow at McGill University) and Brianna Greaves. Kevin Woodger (whose first book is about to appear!) and Jessica Ruffolo took endless photos at the University of Toronto Dental Library. Jessica also created a database of articles that proved extremely useful. Marc-André Gagnon and Curtis Fraser did research in French-language periodicals among the fabulous digital resources of the Bibliothèque et Archives nationales du Québec (BANQ). Melissa Micu provided the inspiration for chapter 6 with her undergraduate thesis on orthodontics and proved to be an outstanding research assistant. She kindly allowed me to use some of our co-written work in this volume. Years ago, Liz Gagnon did research in *Chatelaine*. More recently, Matthew Midolo and Trina Gale expanded on this research to include other women's magazines. Kathryn Hughes helped me with the final edits of this manuscript, and Sarah Campbell helped me review the proofs. I have been very fortunate to work with gifted students over the course of my career – my sincere apologies if I have left anyone out. The funding for all of this student labour was provided by SSHRC and Associated Medical Services: I am very grateful for their support.

Erika Dyck has been a cheerleader for this project, and I am grateful for her encouragement and support. She is a stellar scholar and a model of scholarly generosity. Carlos Quiñonez, a researcher in dental public health at the University of Toronto, has met with me regularly and updated me on changes in the dental world. His outstanding work on dental-public-health history and his contemporary studies of social inequalities and oral health have been an inspiration. Gerodontologist Michael MacEntee met with me in Vancouver and gave me very helpful feedback on chapter 5. Orthodontist William Shaw graciously agreed to my out-of-the-blue e-mail request to read some of what would become chapter 6 and provided excellent advice.

For chapter 2, two scholarly journals kindly allowed me to include parts of previously published articles: the *Canadian Historical Review* (University of Toronto Press): Catherine Carstairs and Rachel Elder, "Expertise, Health and Popular Opinion: Debating Water Fluoridation, 1945–1980," CHR 89, no. 3 (2008): 345–71, doi.org/10.3138/chr.89.3.345; and the *American Journal of Public Health*: Catherine Carstairs, "Debating Water Fluoridation before Dr. Strangelove," AJPH 105, no. 8 (Aug. 2015): 1559–69. For chapter 6, I received the gracious permission of the *Canadian Bulletin of Medical History* (University of Toronto Press) to use parts of Melissa Micu and Catherine Carstairs, "From Improving Egos to Perfecting Smiles: Orthodontics and Psychology, 1945–1990," CBHM 35, no. 2 (2018): 309–36, doi/10.3138/cbmh.237-112017. Other projects are racing to the finish line. Parts of chapters 1 and 3 of *The Smile Gap* will appear in the edited collections *Cultures of Oral Health* (Routledge) and *Medicare's Histories* (University of Manitoba Press), respectively. My sincere thanks to all of these publishers for letting me use all this work.

I've also been able to attend a number of small workshops / conferences where I could share this work. The organizers of the *Medicare at Fifty* conference, University of Winnipeg, September 2018 – Delia Gavrus, James Hanley, and Esyllt Jones – provided me with an opportunity to think through chapter 3. Claire Jones graciously invited me to be part of the Oral Health Humanities and Social Science Network in Britain, and I was able to attend one of its workshops at King's College London, where I received very helpful feedback. In Erin, Ontario, the enthusiasm of the Extended Learning Opportunities Group for the history of cosmetic dentistry and the history of water fluoridation buoyed my spirits and convinced me that there was an audience for this book. The Canadian Historical Association and the Canadian Association of Public Health Dentists allowed me to present parts of chapter 1 at their annual meetings. Kyla Madden at McGill-Queen's University Press expressed interest in this manuscript years ago, but at Congress in Vancouver in June 2019 we talked over the project in detail, and she helped me define the story I wanted to tell, transforming the book in the process. All faults, of course, are mine alone.

THE SMILE GAP

Introduction

Improving Smiles and Creating Gaps

More than a decade ago, I came across a dental report published as part of the Nutrition Canada Survey (1977).[1] Completed in the early 1970s, this was the first extensive study of Canadians' oral health. I was shocked to learn that less than half a century ago, more than 40 per cent of women my age had no teeth in their upper arch, their lower arch, or both arches. Almost a quarter of all adult Canadians had no teeth. I was a toddler in the early 1970s when the Nutrition Canada Survey began, and my oral health experience would be very different. Although I lived in unfluoridated Calgary in my early years, my parents gave me fluoride drops to prevent tooth decay. Later, we moved to fluoridated Winnipeg. Over the course of my life, I have benefitted from fluoridated toothpastes, orthodontic treatment, and regular dental care, except during my years in graduate school when I had no dental insurance. As a result, I have all of my own teeth, except for my wisdom teeth. I've never even had a root canal. My good oral health is partly a consequence of the dramatic changes that have taken place in oral health care since the introduction of water fluoridation in much of urban Canada in the 1950s. But it is also the result of my class and racial privilege, and perhaps a little genetic luck!

I am not alone. On the whole, Canadians enjoy much better oral health than their counterparts did half a century ago. Today, despite the growth of our elderly population, only 6 per cent of Canadians have no teeth, or are edentulous. More than 75 per cent of children aged 6–11 have never had a cavity in their permanent teeth.[2] By comparison, in the mid-1950s, only 33 per cent of children aged 6–8, and fewer than 5 per cent of children aged 9–11, in unfluoridated Sarnia, Ontario, had caries-free permanent teeth.[3] Today, perfect smiles of straight white teeth appear everywhere – in the mouths of my students, on billboards, and in the movies. And yet, real inequalities remain: many people who are disabled, elderly, or living in poverty, and some immigrants, suffer from very poor oral health. Children, especially Indigenous children, continue to undergo surgery requiring anaesthetic for the removal of numerous decayed teeth. Early childhood caries accounts for the largest percentage of day surgeries among children.[4] Rural people still have more difficulty obtaining oral health care than urban residents. People on social assistance, even with dental benefits, often cannot easily locate a dentist who will treat them. Many immigrants see a decline in their oral health after arriving in Canada. Indigenous peoples have much worse oral health than other Canadians, a situation created by a long legacy of austerity in the delivery of health services to them. Ian Mosby and I have explored this in more depth in other publications.[5] I wrote this current book because I wanted to understand and explain how oral health in Canada had so dramatically improved and what this meant for people, especially for those who had not experienced these remarkable gains.

Oral disease leads to bad breath, tooth loss, infection, and pain. It can seriously reduce quality of life. As British dental historian Richard Barnett explains: "Possession of a functional pain-free mouth is a practical necessity – we all must breathe and eat and talk – but it is also central to our sense of self. Pain in the head can seem unbearably close to the core of who we are."[6] Poor oral health can lead to diabetes, strokes and heart attacks, respiratory distress, and low birth weight in babies.[7] But our smiles are also one of the first things we notice about one another. They help to convey who we are. Over the course of the past century, the act of smiling has become an ever-more important aspect of building connection with other people. This is especially important in the service industries. As sociologist Arlie Hochschild showed years ago in her study of airline stewardesses and emotional labour, smiling was a mandatory part of the job.[8] Many service positions require it today. Tooth loss or bad breath can make it difficult to find work. Movie stars, models, and entertainers all have blindingly white, straight teeth, creating new expectations for what our mouths could and should look like. Many people feel unsatisfied with their smiles, and report that crooked and stained teeth shatter their self-esteem.[9] While employers provide dental benefits to many Canadians, this often is not enough to cover the extensive procedures that dentists want to provide and that many patients desire. Dentistry is not just about physical health, it is about beauty, and the ways in which we relate to one another. *The Smile Gap* pays attention not just to oral health, but also to the beauty culture associated with our mouths and teeth.

At the turn of the twentieth century, as I show in chapter 1, Canadians ate diets high in sugar and refined flour and rarely brushed their teeth, leading to an epidemic of tooth decay. At the same time, new theories of tooth decay and its consequences led dentists to stop thinking of themselves as "mechanics of the mouth" and start seeing their roles as medical professionals who understood the biological mechanisms of oral disease. They moved away from conservative dentistry, which focused on repairing the damage caused by tooth decay and concentrated more on prevention. In the early twentieth century, the numbers of dentists in practice skyrocketed, and some began crusading for mouth hygiene. At the same time, an explosion of new media, including the movies, created new expectations for beauty, especially for women. Toothpaste advertising became increasingly aggressive, and full-page ads instructed Canadians on how to care for their teeth and counselled them to smile for success. It seems to be in the first few decades of the twentieth century that many Canadians began to brush their teeth daily – part of a long revolution in personal hygiene that started in the late eighteenth century, as Peter Ward and others have demonstrated.[10]

In the 1930s, American researchers discovered that water supplies with a small amount of naturally occurring fluoride helped prevent tooth decay. As we see in chapter 2, dentists were eager to see if fluorides artificially added to the water supply would do the same. In 1945, Brantford, Ontario, did exactly that in the hope of reducing tooth decay in the city. Immediate results were promising, and in the 1950s, municipalities across Canada began following suit, often in the face of substantial opposition. Many parents in unfluoridated communities began giving their children fluoride tablets or drops. By the early 1960s, the first fluoridated toothpastes became available, leading to further improvements. As provinces expanded their public-health programs, more children and mothers were exposed to oral health education. Together, these interventions would dramatically improve the oral health of Canadians. The famous Crest toothpaste commercials of the 1960s and 1970s – "Look, Ma, no cavities!" – featured smiling children coming home to their parents with positive report cards from the dentists. Such ads were mirroring the truth – cavity rates plummeted across North America in the 1960s and 1970s.

Canadians are incredibly proud of their healthcare system, often citing it as one of the defining features of their national identity. They believe that the Canada Health Act supports Canadian values by providing equal health services to everyone.[11] But the delivery of health care is far from equal, as I explore in chapter 3. Despite the crucial role of oral health in overall well-being, medicare does not cover dentistry. The 1964 *Report of the Royal Commission on Health Services* (Hall Commission), which led to federally funded medicare, recommended free dentistry for all children, and eventually to all adults when there were enough dentists available. Yet this never happened – partly because medicare was proving very expensive, partly because the bulk of dentists opposed the idea, and partly because policy-makers realized that free dental care was potentially regressive: people with the highest incomes tend to use dentists the most, while those with lower incomes are less likely to visit them, even when both groups have access to insurance. A number of provinces did provide dental care to children and to people on social assistance, but some reduced these benefits in the 1980s and 1990s. Access to these benefits can also be very challenging: dentists have often been reimbursed at rates less than their fee schedule to treat people on social assistance, making them unwilling to take on these patients. As well, many were not equipped to treat people with disabilities, and most received little training in this area.

One way to care for underserved groups would be to re-imagine the delivery of dental care. As we see in chapter 3, in Saskatchewan, from 1974 to 1987, dental therapists worked with children in schools, making access much easier for them. Similarly, in many Canadian locales, dental hygienists have delivered mobile care to long-term-care homes. Such auxiliary personnel can improve access to care, but many dentists have pushed to keep all oral health care in private dental offices. Gender plays a central role: most dental therapists and dental hygienists are women. Until very recently, dentistry has been predominantly male, and many practitioners strongly opposed any encroachment on their turf.

While universal dental coverage never became a reality, beginning in the 1970s many Canadians gained access to dental benefits for their families through their employment, as I show in chapter 4. In the 1970s, unions began lobbying hard for dental benefits for their members, partly to make up for the fact that companies no longer needed to provide medical benefits, thanks to the introduction of medicare. Dental coverage also became a way for employers to attract the best professionals and managers. It spread rapidly in the 1970s, and by 2007–09, 62 per cent of Canadians had private coverage.[12] While 32 per cent of Canadians lack coverage, most of those with insurance now visit the dentist frequently, receive regular check-ups and cleaning, and have small problems looked after promptly. Until the explosion of private insurance, many Canadians went to the dentist only when they were in pain, but today the majority visit once or twice a year for check-ups and cleanings. Despite this huge boon for insured people, many working poor do not have dental insurance, with severe consequences for their oral health. Most recent immigrants lack insurance and see their self-reported oral health decline. Certain groups, especially refugees, are particularly likely to suffer from poor oral health in Canada, including caries in early childhood. The disabled often lack care – many dental offices were not accessible until quite recently, and few dentists have appropriate training. While the situation in rural areas has improved since the 1970s, care is often far away, especially from specialists. The expansion of private insurance has improved the oral health of most people but has exacerbated inequalities for those without access to insurance.

Chapter 5 focuses on older adults, a group often left behind by the post-1945 gains. In the 1950s and 1960s, dentists tended to concentrate on children and young adults, regarding older people as a lost cause. By the 1970s, the growing grey power movement, the emergence of gerodontology, and the larger supply of dentists allowed more attention to older patients. Initial studies showed that many senior citizens, especially in old-age homes, badly needed treatment. Most required dentures, many lacked a full set, and others' dentures needed repair and were painful to wear. Over the next few decades, the oral health of seniors began to improve, and more people were keeping their teeth. Even so, serious inequities remain. Retired people are much less likely to have dental benefits than workers. Older people continue to suffer disproportionately from tooth loss and periodontal disease. At the same time, for wealthier Canadians, there are new treatments, most notably dental implants, that can transform people's oral health. While implants are very expensive and not without complications, they provide a much better option than dentures for most people. The massive growth in implants means that inequalities are greater than ever for older Canadians coping with the oral health changes aging may bring.

Just as implants were transforming dentistry for older people, cosmetic dentistry began reshaping Canadians' expectations for their smiles. Chapter 6 reveals that, while orthodontics had long been part of dentistry for more affluent children, in the 1980s growing numbers of adults began sporting braces. The transformation seems to have come about because new technologies were making braces less visible, and because more Canadians could afford adult orthodontics, which was sometimes even partially covered by employer-provided dental benefits. New materials also greatly improved what dentists could offer in terms of caps and veneers. By the 1980s, a number of dentists, often in wealthy neighbourhoods, were describing themselves as "cosmetic dentists," who could transform smiles and create – or so they claimed – happier, more confident patients. The move to cosmetic dentistry exploded at the turn of the century, as the internet and reality television shows made people aware of what cosmetic dentists could accomplish, and intensified people's focus on their appearance. Increasing competition among dentists, and growing debt loads among new dentists, likely also contributed to the growth of cosmetic dentistry. The rise of cosmetic dentistry had made dentistry more than a health service; it is also a beauty service, complicating decisions over what should be covered by public and private insurance.

Historiography

There is a substantial literature on the history of health and illness in Canada, but to date little about the history of dentistry or of oral health. The small literature, both in Canada and internationally, is written mostly by dentists. D.W. Gullett's valuable 1971 historical overview of the profession, written for the Canadian Dental Association, pays little attention to patients or to oral health, and is now very dated.[13] The Ontario Dental Association and the Alberta Dental Association each sponsored commemorative histories.[14] There are histories of dental education at McGill and Dalhousie Universities.[15] Carlos Quiñonez's recent *Politics of Dental Care in Canada* (2021) expertly surveys the political economy of dentistry, including the history of public-health dentistry, while Souad Msefer-Laroussi's 2007 dissertation covers recent publicly funded dental care in Quebec.[16] Tracey L. Adams's fine book on gender, dentistry, and professionalization ends in 1918. Adams argues that dentists emphasized their whiteness and gentlemanliness to appeal to their primarily female patients and bolster their claims to professional privilege and status. In the early twentieth century, dentists began to argue for their profession's scientific status – a claim that would later expand, as this book shows.[17] Adams has also written on interwar female dentists and on the history of dental hygiene, as well as crafting a more recent book on the history of professionalization, in which he includes dentists.[18]

Internationally, Richard Barnett has written a beautifully illustrated history of dental practice, although he devotes only a few pages to the twentieth century; Colin Jones has an insightful book on smiling in eighteenth-century France, and Ruth Roy Harris has a thorough history of the American National Institute of Dental Science.[19] Sarah Nettleton wrote *Power, Pain and Dentistry*, a Foucaultian analysis of dental practice in Britain, with emphasis on the history of dentistry.[20] Like Nettleton,

I explore the disciplinary practices of oral health care: how did many of us come to believe that we should brush our teeth daily and visit a dentist twice each year? Alyssa Picard's excellent *Making the American Mouth: Dentists and Public Health in the Twentieth Century* embeds the history of oral health, dentistry, and social inequality in social, cultural, and political history, with a focus on dentistry and American identity.[21]

This book is influenced by the move towards patient-oriented history. In the late 1970s, medical history underwent a "social turn," moving away from the history of discovery and of great men paying more attention to the gender, racial, and class dynamics of health care and the history of patients.[22] In Canada, this resulted in books like Geoffrey Bilson's *A Darkened House*, Wendy Mitchinson's *The Nature of Their Bodies*, and Rosemary and David Gagan's *For Patients of Moderate Means*.[23] This trend has continued and is still thriving more than four decades later. Recent outstanding examples include Maureen Lux's *Separate Beds*, Esyllt Jones's *Influenza 1918*, and Erika Dyck's *Facing Eugenics*.[24] While the available sources did not allow me to write the current volume as an entirely patient-focused history, I tried to include the voices of patients whenever possible.

This volume adds to the growing literature on medicare and health insurance in Canada. Despite popular reverence for medicare and the importance of health services to our lives and deaths, the literature remains small. It includes classic texts by David Naylor and Malcolm Taylor, as well as a more recent edited volume by Gregory Marchildon and a forthcoming collection edited by Delia Gavrus, James Hanley, and Esyllt Jones.[25] Political scientists Gerard Boychuk and Antonia Maioni have provided very useful US–Canadian comparisons.[26] Esyllt Jones's *Radical Medicine* offers a fascinating look at the transnational influences on Saskatchewan's innovative health-care initiatives in the post-1945 era.[27] Dentistry, of course, is not part of medicare, and this book has been influenced by Beatrix Hoffman's outstanding monograph on American medical rationing, which argues that health care has always been rationed, usually by ability to pay, and sometimes by notions of who was "deserving" of care, despite passionate pleas against rationing by opponents of "Obamacare" and the Clinton proposals for reforming health care. Similar patterns shape the provision of oral health care in Canada.[28]

This book makes an important contribution to the history of health professions. There is a notable literature on medicine and nursing, but the other health professions in English-speaking Canada have been neglected, except for valuable work by Peter Twohig on laboratory workers, Ivy Lynn Bourgeault and Megan Davies on midwives, Ruby

Heap on physiotherapy, and Sasha Mullally on occupational therapy.[29] In Quebec, the history of health professions is much more fully developed, with excellent work on audiology, dietetics, occupational therapy, and physiotherapy.[30] There is a rich social-science literature on the health professions by scholars such as Patricia O'Reilly and Tracey Adams that pays close attention to the process of professionalization.[31] Except for Adams's excellent work on the professionalization of dentistry and recent history of dental hygiene, scholars have not yet examined the history of the oral health professions.[32] In chapter 5, I explore the story of denturists (once known as dental mechanics), an atypically male-dominated health profession. This book also adds to the history of dentistry, of dental therapy (previously known as dental nursing), and of dental hygiene, although I explored the last in more depth in an article in *Gender and History*.[33]

This book is shaped by the growing body of literature on the social determinants of health. Over the past quarter-century, epidemiologists have emphasized that even in wealthy countries with universal health care, like Canada, wealthier people live significantly longer and suffer fewer illnesses than the poor. Inequality starts in the womb. Women who live in poverty during their pregnancies cannot afford to eat as well and often receive inadequate prenatal care. Poor fetal development affects a person's entire life course. Parents with higher levels of education are more likely to have the income and the time required to exercise and to eat well, so their offspring are more likely to eat nutritiously and engage in sports and healthy recreation. Children who enter school with lower vocabularies see these effects magnified – they are less likely to become well-educated, their employment prospects are worse, and at all stages of life they are more likely to experience ill-health. The degree of people's control over their work also influences health: coronary heart disease, for example, is nearly twice as high in people who report having a low level of control at work. Stress strongly affects health: it weakens the immune system and leads to increased insulin resistance and lipid and clotting disorders. The fear of eviction, food insecurity, and job losses are all notable sources of stress. People living in poverty are more vulnerable to the devastating impacts of addiction to drugs and alcohol, which they may use to blunt the demoralizing effects of poverty. They are more likely to eat more refined, high-calorie foods, because they are cheaper than fresh fruits and vegetables and more readily available in poor neighbourhooods. As a result, they are more likely to consume an excess of calories, which can lead to cardiovascular disease, cancer, and diabetes. We know that social isolation, low self-esteem, and anxiety can make people vulnerable to infections and lead to diabetes, high blood pressure, heart attacks, and strokes. There is also substantial research that shows that racism affects health in multiple ways: systemic racism means that BIPOC (Black, Indigenous, and People of Colour) individuals are more likely to live in disadvantaged neighbourhoods, have lower levels of education, and have less control over their work, while micro-aggressions and overt racism contribute to higher levels of stress and disease.[34] As this book shows, the social determinants of health are especially obvious in oral health.

There is a larger story to tell about racism and dentistry that I hope other scholars will explore in more detail. Unfortunately, my attempts to interview BIPOC dentists were not successful. A patient's perspective on this issue would also be a vital addition. An emerging literature on race and health equity in Canada suggests that much more research needs to be done on the health impacts of racism.[35] Ideas about race have shaped research in the dental field; racism affects how dentists treat their patients and has influenced who gets to be a dentist or oral health professional. From the mid-nineteenth century onwards, dental researchers were interested in racial differences in mouth shape and dentition. Some, such as the Canadian dentist Weston Price, a leading dental figure in the first half of the twentieth century, were interested in racial differences in oral health, usually positing that so-called primitive peoples had much healthier dentition than so-called civilized people. This undoubtedly affected how dentists approached their patients.[36] More recently, significant literature has emerged, as I discuss in chapter 4, on immigrants and access to oral health and oral health care, but that work addresses immigration status more than racism and covers only the very recent past.

Racism also affects who enters the field of dentistry. After a shockingly misogynistic Facebook group was uncovered among male students at Dalhousie University, *The Report of the Task Force on Misogyny, Sexism and Homophobia* in the university's Faculty of Dentistry depicted a long history of racism, homophobia, and misogyny at the school.[37] This was not a problem not just at Dalhousie. Throughout Canada, many BIPOC dentists faced racial discrimination. Wah Leung, the founding dean of the University of British Columbia (UBC) Dental School, appointed in 1962, grew up in Vancouver and completed his DDS at McGill but was banned from practising in British Columbia. He moved to the United States, where he established a successful career before being invited back to UBC.[38] Sunny Lee, a Victoria-born dentist, also graduated from McGill, but when he moved to Vancouver in the late 1940s, he had to borrow money from his family to set up his dental office in downtown

Vancouver, as the banks refused him a loan.[39] Despite the racial barriers, visible minorities may have found dentistry slightly more welcoming than medicine, given that dental schools were worried about a lack of well-qualified applicants until the 1970s, and dentists, unlike physicians, do not need to do a residency, which was often a significant obstacle for Jews and visible minorities in medicine, as hospitals were loath to employ them as residents.[40] Things started to change in the 1970s, when immigration to Canada became more diverse, and overt discrimination became less socially acceptable. By the 1970s, the Faculty of Dentistry at the University of Toronto was attracting significant numbers of Asian students, although Black students were far less common and Indigenous students non-existent.[41]

Research from the United States shows that the race of caregivers can affect health outcomes of racialized patients.[42] It is hard to know how the diversification of dentistry changed patient care, especially since some minority groups were still poorly represented and because it can be very hard to achieve change when you are one of the first to enter a field. Senator Mary Jane McCallum, from Barren Lands First Nation, was the first Indigenous dentist in Canada, graduating from the University of Manitoba in 1990. In an interview with the alumni magazine, she reported that she initially delivered care in a "rigid, Westernized approach" and that it took some time for her to take a more holistic, Indigenous approach to her patients.[43] This shows why it is vital to have dentists of all backgrounds, as well as historians of all backgrounds to explore the history of dentistry.

I intend this study to be, as much as possible, a national history. There is a heavy focus on Ontario, the most populated province, home to the country's largest dental school, and a centre of dental research and policy-making. Ontario was also a pioneer in public dental health in the early twentieth century. Saskatchewan also figured largely, with the nation's most innovative oral health policies in the years after 1945 and a rich archival record. Some of the most valuable research on poverty and oral health has been done by researchers at the Université de Montréal, and superb materials are available at the Bibliothèque et Archives nationales du Québec (BANQ). Other provinces appear in the story when sources supported their inclusion.

This book relies on a range of sources. The archival record is thin. Don Gullett, the long-time secretary of the Canadian Dental Association (CDA), and the author of the most complete history of dentistry in Canada, arranged for the CDA to donate the papers he used for his book to Library and Archives Canada, but these are very heavy on institutional history and end in the late 1970s. I also reviewed the records of the Dental Division within the federal Department of National Health and Welfare. The invaluable records in Regina, Saskatchewan, include those of the Saskatchewan Dental Therapists Association and the Saskatchewan Dental Hygiene Association. I supplemented this with material from the Toronto and Vancouver city archives on municipal dental-health programs.

More useful even than archival sources were government reports. I examined the annual reports of National Health and Welfare's Dental Division, as well as provincial reports from British Columbia, Nova Scotia, Ontario, and Quebec. The Canadian government undertook major surveys of dental health, including *The Canadian Sickness Survey* (1951), Nutrition Canada's *Dental Survey* (1977), and *The Canadian Health Measures Survey* (2010). The Royal Commission on Health Services (Hall Commission) produced several very useful volumes, including Bruce A. McFarlane's *Dental Manpower in Canada* (1965) and K.J. Paynter's *Dental Education in Canada* (1965). I explored Hansard for parliamentary debates, as well as records of legislative debates in Ontario and Quebec. I also examined pamphlets and films used to educate people on how to care for their teeth, as well as school hygiene textbooks.

I undertook much of my research at the Dentistry Library at the University of Toronto. The *Journal of the Canadian Dental Association* (*JCDA*), the voice of organized dentistry in the country, was particularly helpful. I went through every volume in the period under examination here and had a research assistant index and tag every article. It provided me with an excellent overview of research in dentistry, curricular changes at dental faculties across the country, shifts in the economics of dental practice, trends in practice management, and issues that concerned dentists, from dreaded "state dentistry" in the 1940s to battles with insurance companies in the 1970s and 1980s. The *JCDA* also allowed me to look at the care of certain underserved groups, such as children, the elderly, and people on social assistance. By the 1970s, the dental literature was increasingly international, and as a result, I looked more at the international research literature, doing searches in PubMed and cross-referencing with Google Scholar to determine which articles had had the biggest influence in the field. I also made extensive use of dental textbooks. As well, I used the *Canadian Public Health Association Journal*, the *Dominion Dental Journal*, *Oral Health*, and *Transactions of the Canadian Dental Association*. Another invaluable source was the *Canadian Dental Hygiene Journal*, which was renamed *Probe* in 1986. Dental hygienists have traditionally concentrated on education and patient care and were conscious and often critical of their subservient position in the dental office. Their journal provided a different perspective on oral health care than the dentistry journals.

The popular press, including magazines and newspapers, was an incredibly valuable source for understanding how expectations for smiles changed over time. In *Chatelaine*, the *Canadian Home Journal*, and *Revue moderne*, I paid close attention to advertisements for oral hygiene products as well as articles instructing women how to care for their own and their children's teeth. I carefully examined covers to see how expectations of smiling have changed. I made full use of newspapers across the country, including the incredible resources that now exist through BANQ and newspapers.com. *Benefits Canada*, a periodical devoted to personnel benefits, was very revealing on the history of dental insurance. I also found myself looking at some unexpected sources, like yellow-page ads, etiquette guides, and television makeover shows.

At the beginning of this project, I intended to do extensive oral interviews. As it turns out, it was hard to find dentists who were willing to talk to me. Most of those who were were female practitioners whom I contacted when I was doing research for a paper on women in dentistry. The Canadian Dental Hygiene Association was incredibly generous and put me in touch with many of its leaders. I did fourteen interviews with dental hygienists. Although I was tempted by the idea of interviewing patients, a mock interview with a friend had her breaking down in tears, underlining how strongly people feel about the appearance of their teeth and mouth. I decided that I did not have the training or resources to do interviews that were potentially traumatic for either party. Instead, I relied on published accounts in newspapers and academic journals.

While my focus is on Canada, its dentists had close ties to their American counterparts. Many attended US undergraduate schools, especially before dental education in Canada expanded in the 1960s. Specialists and faculty members had frequently done advanced training in the United States. They read the American journals and relied on American textbooks. When continuing education became more common for dentists, they frequently travelled to the United States, sometimes to link continuing education with skiing or golf.[44] In comparison to Canadian medical practice, which under medicare became very different from American, dentistry remained very similar in the two countries. Many Canadian dental patients learned how to take care of their mouths from US ads and media. Accordingly, I also examined American debates, sources, and stories that were influential in Canada. British dentistry had far less impact, but I have incorporated material from Britain where relevant. After the United States, Canadian dentists talked most about

New Zealand, which pioneered a children's dental service that would be copied by Saskatchewan and widely discussed elsewhere in Canada.

This is the first history of oral health in Canada. I hope it will not be the last. Oral health affects how we smile, how we laugh, and how we engage with the world. It appears to play a role in cardiovascular disease, diabetes, low birth weights, and other chronic health conditions. While Canadians have learned a great deal about how to care for their teeth over the past century, many still lack access to necessary dental care. I hope that this book will underline the importance of having a more equitable system of care for everyone.

1

Learning to Smile

Oral Health Education, Advertising, and Brushing

In 1910, the Toronto Board of Education hired Dr William Doherty, a demonstrator and teacher at the Royal College of Dental Surgeons of Ontario, to inspect the teeth of the city's schoolchildren. He examined 643, only 70 of whom reported brushing their teeth daily.[1] At the Elizabeth Street School in the working-class Ward district, 76 per cent could not chew properly, 61 per cent had abscesses in their mouth, 45 per cent had pus exuding into their mouth, 47 per cent had enlarged salivary glands, and 87 per cent had poor oral hygiene. Forty-two per cent were suffering from toothache at the time of examination.[2] At the more affluent Church Street School, conditions were considerably better. Even so, 55 per cent of the youngsters could not chew properly, 21 per cent had abscesses, 16 per cent were exuding pus, and 56 per cent had poor oral hygiene. Twenty-two per cent had toothaches when Doherty examined them. He summarized: "The menace in the decay and loss of the teeth on the health of school children is manifold. It renders thorough mastication impossible and establishes the habit of bolting the food, while the filth which is inseparable from decaying, putrescent and abscessed teeth, is mixed with the food and carried to the stomach." He complained: "Gastro-intestinal disorders, anemia, toxemia, and malnutrition are some of the more obvious results, lowering the vital potential of the child and making it a ready victim of other and more serious diseases."[3] It seems that adult mouths in Canada were not much better. According to a *Maclean's* article from 1910, "even with good care and conservative dentistry, it is unusual to keep natural teeth comfortable and useful much beyond the age of fifty."[4]

It is not surprising that people's teeth were such a mess – in the late nineteenth century and into the twentieth, skyrocketing consumption of sugar and refined carbohydrates was generating an epidemic of tooth decay.[5] Few children had ever seen a dentist, and it is likely that only a fraction regularly brushed their teeth. Over the next few decades, the situation would change: an invigorated dental profession would draw attention to the links between oral health and the health of the rest of the body, while advertisers selling toothpaste and toothbrushes informed consumers of the need to brush their teeth regularly. A new emphasis on beauty, created in part by better photography in magazines and the introduction of motion pictures, created a demand for charming smiles, especially for women.[6] Schools across the country began teaching oral hygiene, and in some cities children's teeth were inspected regularly. The toothbrushing stampede was part of a larger revolution in self-care, which Mariana Valverde has described in *The Age of Light, Soap, and Water*.[7] As Nancy Tomes detailed in the *Gospel of Germs*, about the turn of the twentieth century, Americans (and, I would argue, Canadians) absorbed the lessons of germ theory and embraced rituals of germ-avoidance to improve their own health and their children's.[8] Brushing teeth was one of these rituals. It was not unknown in the nineteenth century, but in the 1910s and 1920s what African-American reformer Booker T. Washington described as the "gospel of the toothbrush" took hold.[9]

Why Were People's Teeth So Bad?

Dental caries is a disease largely of diet. Foods rich in sugar and starch feed the bacteria that produce acids that attack tooth enamel. During the nineteenth century, Canadian foodways changed: industrial milling of flour produced bread that was cheaper, less nutritious, and richer in carbohydrates than whole-grain breads. As people moved into towns and cities, opportunities to eat fresh fruit and vegetables diminished. The growth of Caribbean sugar plantations made refined sugar cheaper and more accessible.[10] As Bettina Bradbury discovered for industrializing Montreal, families survived primarily on bread, sugar, tea, coffee, oatmeal, and rice. Vegetables and apples were available in summer, and some families kept chickens.[11] According to Bradbury, "Bread was the working-class staple food."[12] Little had likely changed by 1912, when University of Toronto researcher H.B. Anderson showed how many calories derived from 25 cents' worth of various foodstuffs: bread, sugar, potatoes, and oatmeal delivered the most calories, and meats, eggs, and cheese the fewest. Potatoes were the only "vegetables" Anderson costed, an indication of the limited role of vegetables in Torontonian diets at the time.[13]

In short, most people were consuming highly cariogenic foods. As Caroline Durand has persuasively argued, the quality of diets of "*les gens de classes modestes*" actually declined in the years before the Great War.[14] W. Peter Ward and Patricia Ward showed that the weight of children born to poor Montreal mothers decreased between 1851 and 1905, probably because of the mothers' poor diets.[15] Similarly, John Cranfield and Kris Inwood have shown that men born after 1894 were shorter than those born in the 1870s, suggesting that the quality and sufficiency of food may have been declining, although this was not the only factor at play.[16] At least 20 per cent of the recipes in *The Five Roses Cookbook* (1915), Canada's most popular recipe book of the era, were for cake, and 40 per cent were for pies, pudding, cookies, biscuits, tarts, buns, rolls, and bread. There was no vegetable category. While the focus on white flour had much to do with the corporate creator of the cookbook (a milling company), the fact that the collection was such a success indicates that Canadians greatly enjoyed these foods.[17] Dental researcher Aubrey Sheiham demonstrated similar trends for Britain, where a dramatic increase in dental caries began in the late nineteenth century and continued through the early twentieth, coinciding with a rise in sugar consumption.[18]

The discovery of various vitamins (A, B1, B2, C, D, and E between 1910 and 1922 and many others in the 1920s and 1930s) led many nutritionists and other health professionals to stress consumption of "the protective foods," including milk and leafy vegetables.[19] Even so, consumption of sugar and carbohydrates remained high in Canada, falling off only after the Second World War, which brought increased attention to the importance of a balanced diet.[20] In 1943, a survey asking schoolchildren aged 10–14 in Quebec what they had eaten in the previous 24 hours found that 50 per cent had consumed only white bread, highly refined cereals, meat, potatoes, pastry, and sweets.[21] Statistics Canada surveys of households' food expenditures showed that sugar provided 12.6 per cent of a typical household's energy in 1938–39, but only 7.9 per cent in 1953, and 6.1 per cent in 1969. Likewise, store-bought bread provided 19.4 per cent in 1938–39 and only 14.8 per cent in 1953, revealing that in the interwar years people were eating a diet that predisposed them to tooth decay and tooth loss.[22] But other factors helped generate poor dental health: treatment was costly, many people feared low-speed drills, and dentists were still trying to figure out how to go beyond repairing damaged teeth to preventing tooth decay.

Dentistry

The professionalization of dentistry began in France with the work of Pierre Fauchard (1679–1761), the so-called father of dentistry. His famous text, *Le chirurgien dentiste* (1728), detailed how to remove the carious parts of the tooth and fill it with lead or tin. He described how to construct bridges and dentures using human teeth or ivory, as well as spring devices to keep the dentures in place. He argued for keeping the mouth clean, including using a mouthwash of one's own urine.[23] In the nineteenth century, Americans led the way, setting up the first professional association (the American Society of Dental Surgeons, founded 1839), the first professional journal (the *American Journal of Dental Science*, 1840), and the first formal school of dentistry (the Baltimore College of Dental Surgery, also 1840). Professional dentistry moved more slowly in Canada. The first sustained professional journal, the *Dominion Dental Journal*, was established in 1889, with W. George Beers as editor. Beers (1843–1900) is well known for his sporting activities, including appropriating the Iroquois game of lacrosse for settler Canadians, but he was also the most noted dentist of his era, serving as president of the Quebec Dental Association and dean of the Dental College of the Province of Quebec.[24] In Toronto in 1875, the Royal College of Dental Surgeons of Ontario created Canada's first dental school, which affiliated with the University of Toronto in 1889 but did not join it formally until 1925. The Dental College of the Province of Quebec came into being in 1892, offering degrees from Bishop's University, which then had a medical school in Montreal. The medical school was dissolved in 1905, and dental education was turned over to Laval University's Montreal campus, later the Université de Montréal, and to McGill University.[25] The Maritime Dental College in Halifax began accepting students in 1908, offering degrees conferred by Dalhousie University.[26] The University of Alberta, in Edmonton, would become Canada's fourth dental school when it launched a dental course in 1918. Ontario's Royal College was much larger than the other schools and was the dominant force in dental education and research in Canada.

Despite these moves to professionalize dentistry, many Canadian practitioners had little formal training. As late as 1909, when the first national directory appeared, well under half of the western contingent had DDS degrees. In Ontario, 70 per cent did, and 53 per cent in Quebec.[27] To the dismay of organized practitioners, probably the best-known Canadian dentist of the era was Edgar Randolph Parker (1872–1952), or "Painless Parker" – he officially changed his name after new regulations in California forbade him from advertising painless dentistry. Parker was born in rural New Brunswick. After being expelled from Acadia University for bad behaviour, he worked as a sailor and as a travelling salesman: he would put these sales skills to work as a dentist. His unhappy parents gave him the money to attend the New York College of Dentistry. He finished his degree at the Philadelphia Dental College and returned home, hoping for a career in New Brunswick. His practice was a failure until a friend told him that people were afraid of dentists, so he moved to a neighbouring town and renamed himself "Painless Parker – the Great Dentist." He borrowed a wagon and recruited an audience with a dinner horn, promising to extract teeth without pain. Soon he was making money and taking his show across the country. He was reportedly one of the first dentists to use cocaine as a topical anaesthetic. Wearing a top hat and a necklace of extracted teeth, he would take out teeth in front of an audience that was being entertained by a brass band, contortionists, and dancers. After a few attempts at a more standard practice, he set up a very successful dental circus that criss-crossed the continent. He would sometimes pull the teeth of lions or tigers to gain publicity. Eventually, he relocated to California, where he set up a chain of offices along the west coast, including one in Vancouver. He continued to do battle with professional dentistry, which abhorred his publicity stunts, but he did very well into the 1930s. A movie based loosely on his life, featuring Jane Russell and Bob Hope, was made in 1948.[28] Parker was not alone in practising outside the approval of organized dentistry: classified newspaper ads suggested learning from the BC School of Mechanical Dentistry, which earned the profession's ire.[29]

Painless Parker's profitable antics aside, dentistry was progressing in the late nineteenth and early twentieth centuries. Dentists are proud that it was one of their own, Horace Wells, who initiated the use of nitrous oxide (laughing gas) in medicine in the 1840s. Use of ether and chloroform followed quickly, although general anaesthesia was not without risk and was generally reserved for serious operations. Dentists also used cocaine for topical freezing, but it was highly addictive. Novocain, introduced in the early twentieth century, was a notable breakthrough, making dentistry far less uncomfortable.[30] X-rays allowed more accurate diagnosis, though not without danger for dentists or patients.[31] Many practitioners took private courses in radiology in the 1910s and 1920s.[32] Many also embraced germ theory and became convinced that "mouth hygiene" could significantly improve oral health.

In 1890, W.D. Miller, an American dentist inspired by the bacteriologist Robert Koch, published *Micro-organisms of the Human Mouth*, which argued that tooth decay was a two-part process. First, acid left by food residues dissolved the tooth enamel; then micro-organisms attacked the inner layers of the tooth. Miller's work inspired a "mouth hygiene" movement that urged people to brush their teeth, just as public-health campaigns were promoting spotless homes, open windows, and clean children.[33] In Toronto, leading dentists formed the Canadian Oral Prophylactic Association (COPA) in 1905 to design a useful toothpaste. The founders believed that many available preparations were "positively harmful," as they contained starches and sugars. At first, they distributed their formula to dentists to prescribe for their patients, but this required compounding it at a pharmacy, which was inconvenient, so they sought a manufacturer. They called their toothpaste "Hutax" and kept adjusting its formula in the light of new information and poured the profits into oral hygiene education.[34] The product was not advertised until the early 1930s, when production was turned over to the McGillvary Company. Due to the Depression and the highly competitive market, McGillvary struggled to sell the toothpaste and eventually the COPA dissolved, but not before it became a force in oral health education, distributing toothbrushes and toothpastes, sponsoring lectures to schools and community groups, and urging dentists to push for preventive mouth and dental care.[35]

In 1911, Wallace Secombe, a leading dentist, started the journal *Oral Health*, which was distributed free to all dentists in Canada, propagating oral hygiene. Thanks to these advances in the science of dentistry and growing professionalization, in the 1910s and 1920s dentists began to see themselves as medical professionals who worked to save teeth and improve health.[36] They started to shift emphasis from the mechanical work of constructing dentures, filling teeth, and building crowns and bridges to prevention of tooth decay altogether. As the president of the Ontario Dental Association explained in 1912, "The great work of our profession must be along the lines of prevention rather than correction or repair. This work must have its origin in the education of the people to realize the great importance of their teeth."[37] As Tracey L. Adams shows, dentists began to value mouth health as part of overall health, claiming that neglect of it could lead to insanity, chronic illness, and moral and physical degeneracy.[38] In their professional journals, dentists urged brushing the teeth at least twice a day (after every meal was regarded as preferable but impractical) and proposed various methods of brushing.[39] In the United States, Alfred Fones established the profession of dental hygiene, and his *Mouth Hygiene* (1916) became the standard reference.[40]

These various developments had an impact: school textbooks began to include more information on the importance of cleaning the teeth and detailed instructions for how to do so. The hygiene guide for schools and colleges prepared by the Provincial Board of Health of Ontario in 1886 recommended cleaning the teeth with a toothbrush but provided no specific instructions.[41] A Quebec counterpart (1891) stressed looking after teeth, but suggested only "washing" them with fresh water or a powder dentifrice.[42] A later Quebec guide (1906) urged brushing every morning, rinsing after every meal, and using a tooth powder three times a week.[43] *Hygiene for Young People* (1911), the recommended text in Ontario for students in form III (approximately today's grade 6),[44] proposed cleaning food residues off teeth with a quill toothpick and toothbrush, lest "small plants" grow on the teeth, invisible to the naked eye but able to thrive in the warm, moist mouth, just as summer's heat and rain generate flowers, and these plants would produce acid that would lead to tooth decay. The manual recommended brushing up and down and using a tooth powder, followed by a mouthwash like Listerine.[45] *Scouting for Boys* (1908), outsold apparently by only the Bible in the years before the Second World War, also urged twice-daily brushing.[46]

Focal Infection

The campaign for prevention and mouth hygiene was greatly aided by the theory of focal infection.[47] Experts had long claimed that infections in the mouth could lead to illness elsewhere in the body. Hippocrates claimed to cure a case of arthritis by removing a tooth. So did the famed American physician Benjamin Rush.[48] The theory was re-invigorated in 1900 by the British surgeon William Hunter, who claimed in the *British Medical Journal* that "the constant swallowing of pus" was "a most potent and prevalent cause of gastric trouble." He suggested oral sepsis as a cause of tonsillitis, ulcerative endocarditis, meningitis, osteomyelitis, and other conditions. He recommended removal of all dead teeth, vigorous daily sterilizing of dental plates, and avoidance of "conservative dentistry," such as bridges, that could not be kept sterile.[49] At a lecture at McGill University in 1910 that helped bring his theory to the attention of Canadian doctors and dentists, he asserted that he admired the "sheer ingenuity and mechanical skill" of dental surgeons, but added that their work created "ghastly tragedies." He claimed that the "worst cases of anaemia, gastritis, colitis ... nervous disturbances of all kinds ... chronic rheumatic affections" and kidney disease were caused by construction of "a veritable mausoleum of gold fillings, crowns and bridges over a mass of sepsis."[50] This lecture was subsequently published in the prestigious medical journal the *Lancet*. In 1912, Frank Billings, dean of the

University of Chicago's Medical School and a former president of the American Medical Association, argued that chronic focal infections led to arthritis and nephritis. He further promulgated this theory in a series of lectures at Stanford in 1915.[51] At the legendary Mayo Clinic in Rochester, Minnesota, E.C. Rosenow carried out a series of experiments extracting streptococci from people and injecting the bacteria into animals. He concluded that infections in the mouth could lead to arthritis and heart disease.[52] The most-used textbook of the era, Russell Cecil's *Textbook of Medicine* (1928), had a chapter on focal infections that claimed they were the cause of arthritis, nephritis, neuralgias, and general debility, including gastro-intestinal distress. He recommended removing the primary focus – usually tonsils or teeth. He suggested X-rays of the teeth before removal and extracting only one or two teeth at first – and the others two weeks later.[53]

Another major advocate of focal infections was Dr Weston Price, a Canadian-born dentist turned researcher, whose *Nutrition and Physical Degeneration* (1939) continues to be well-cited in alternative nutrition circles today. In 1916, the COPA invited him to speak in Toronto, where he attracted a large audience of physicians and dentists; the printed address was much cited in the years to come.[54] Price had just heard Dr Charles Mayo (the famed surgeon and a founder of the eponymous clinic) speak in Chicago. Mayo maintained that the era of epidemic disease was coming to an end. Instead, he claimed 90 per cent of people would die of a simple infection, caused in most cases by a focal infection, usually originating in the mouth. Price urged dentists to do further research on focal infections and to cooperate with their medical colleagues, as he felt that physicians were ordering removal of too many teeth. They needed dentists to help them understand which teeth might be the cause of infection and which could safely remain in the mouth. And yet, he acknowledged, "a lot of my dental operations have helped to shorten the lives of patients."[55] Foreshadowing his subsequent work on nutrition, he concluded, "I have no hesitation in saying that the Cliff Dwellers with their healthy mouths without decay were infinitely better off than our civilization with our boasted dentistry, because we do now know better than to hitch sick teeth on well teeth."[56] Price later published a book on focal infections.[57]

Dentists used the theory to make their case for mouth health. According to dentist F.J. Conboy, director of Dental Services for Ontario's Provincial Board of Health and later mayor of Toronto, "There appears to be no escape from the conclusion that many of the degenerative diseases which appear to be on the increase, have as one of their important, and in many cases their chief causative factor, dental infection."[58]

Nova Scotia dentist H.W. Black claimed in the *Public Health Journal* that focal infection and pyorrhoea (gum disease) might be the "actual or contributing cause of such dreaded diseases as Brights, Diabetes, Gall Bladder, Gastric Ulcers, Anaemia, Rheumatism, Pericarditis and Endocarditis, Auto-intoxication, Nervous prostration, Sciatica, Neuraliga, Neuritis, Artea Sclorosis, Goiter, Epilepsy, Insanity, Consumption, Facial Erruptions and numerous other disquieting dangerous or disfiguring disorders."[59] He quoted Dr Irons, a heart specialist in Chicago, as saying that half of all US deaths from heart disease were "due to diseased teeth," while Dr Cotton, superintendent of the State Hospital for the Insane in Trenton, New Jersey, claimed that half of the asylum's patients were there because of abscessed teeth.[60]

Doctors were convinced and began taking mouth health more seriously, though they were often very critical of dentists for having created the problem in the first place with all their crowns and bridges. Sir William Osler's famed textbook, *Principles and Practices of Medicine* (1923), paid homage to Hunter and suggested monthly cleaning of teeth by a dentist.[61] A cover article in the *Canadian Medical Association Journal* in July 1920 claimed: "Dental focal infections are very common, more so now than years ago, and because of the progress of dental science. This paradox is explained by the increase in so-called conservative dentistry. Aching, decayed, dead or infected teeth were formerly extracted. During the last twenty years, especially in city dwellers, these teeth are preserved to the patients by treatment filling the root canals and covering them up with gold crowns. 'Uneasy lies the tooth that wears a crown.'"[62] The author claimed that dental infection was the cause of genito-urinary tract infections, goiter, Hodgkin's Disease, hypertension, phlebitis, rheumatism, septicaemia, and ulcers.[63]

Dentists retorted that many physicians were being swept along by the theory, urging extraction of salvageable teeth. At a joint meeting of the Medical Society of Nova Scotia and the Halifax Dental Association, Dr J.S. Bagnall of the Faculty of Dentistry at Dalhousie urged doctors to consider the illness's severity, the patient's natural defences, X-rays, possible treatment of the tooth, and extraction's effect on mastication. "Sacrifice of teeth without due consideration of possible results is to be deplored."[64] Similarly, at a meeting of the Ontario Dental Association, Chicago dentist C.H. Johnston, a graduate of Ontario's Royal College, lambasted doctors and dentists for "alleged recklessness in depriving long-suffering humanity of its instruments of mastication." He concluded, "We have been stampeded out of our sanity by a hue and cry of focal infection." He urged physicians to consult with dentists before ordering tooth extractions.[65]

The theory was also well-known to members of the public. During his brief time in Toronto in the early 1920s, Ernest Hemingway wrote an article for the *Toronto Star Weekly* on "one hundred percenters" – dentists who pulled every tooth with an infected root. He sided with conservative dentists who did not pull every infected tooth, condemning the 100 percenters as a fad.[66] Through the 1910s and 1920s, newspapers ran regular articles on focal infection, while doctors and dentists lectured on the phenomenon.[67] For example, in 1920, dentist Dr Winthrope in Saskatchewan addressed the local Kiwanis Club; his speech generated a newspaper article as well. He claimed that dentistry had focused on repairing teeth but now sought to put "a patient's mouth in a condition of perfect cleanliness." He cited Charles Mayo's claim that "90 percent of all deaths in civilized countries would be caused by focal infection."[68] At Convocation Hall, University of Toronto, in 1928, Mayo himself insisted that focal infections caused many degenerative diseases.[69] As one dentist stated in the *JCDA*, "The average well-informed individual is cognizant of the systemic disturbances resultant from dental disorders."[70]

The theory of focal infection was never fully accepted and lasted but a few decades. By 1940, studies were showing unpredictable results: many patients with indigestion worsened when their teeth were removed.[71] Psychiatric ailments returned. The theory fell out of favour, but, while it held sway, it helped convince many dentists to look more to prevention, to acquire better training in the biological sciences, and do more research.[72] It also spurred many doctors and dentists to work together.[73] The acknowledgment that mouth health and overall well-being were deeply connected fuelled the growth of oral hygiene education across Canada. The Canadian Dental Hygiene Council (CDHC), a group of dentists and laymen, was founded in 1924 with the support of the Canadian Dental Association and its provincial counterparts. With funding from the Dominion government, the Canadian Life Insurance Officer's Association, and the COPA (which turned over its oral hygiene activities to the CDHC), the CDHC carried out campaigns for dental hygiene in various provinces: it focused on Saskatchewan (1927–28), Manitoba (1928–29), Alberta (1929–30), and British Columbia and Quebec (1930–31). In Saskatchewan, it contacted medical officers of health across the province, asking them to speak on mouth health, printed 25,000 booklets in English and 10,000 in Ukrainian, and set up free dental clinics in hospitals across the province.[74] In British Columbia in 1930–31, it showed films on "mouth health" at cinemas, conducted dental examinations across the province, launched a free travelling clinic, and distributed literature to students and teachers.[75] In Manitoba, a Canadian Foundation for Preventive Dentistry arranged for talks on radio stations and a travelling dental clinic to rural areas.[76] In 1935, all the schoolchildren in Charlottetown, Prince Edward Island, had their teeth inspected, and the CDHC gave talks on oral hygiene at every school.[77] The last province to be covered was Nova Scotia in 1937–38. Its Department of Health distributed 40,000 copies of CDHC literature. Every dentist in the province gave up two days that year to inspect children's teeth – charts were made in duplicate, one for the child's home, one for the school nurse. In four towns, dental treatment was arranged for needy children, with men's service clubs paying. Lectures on dental health were given to school groups and service associations in 22 communities.[78]

In the mid-1920s, the Ontario Dental Association produced two pamphlets, *The Treasure House* (for youngsters) and *Joy of Living* (for older children and parents), which the CDHC distributed across the country.[79] The fanciful *Treasure House* urged younger children to think of themselves as a castle, their mouths as the entrance, and their teeth as the guards. To protect their teeth, they needed to eat healthy foods, including milk, eggs, fruit, cheese, vegetables, and coarse bread. The pamphlet warned that sugar and candy led to tooth decay. It urged children to brush their teeth four times a day – once after each meal and once before bedtime.[80] (Such frequent brushing was a constant in the instructive literature from the 1920s to the 1970s, as dentists believed that tooth decay started almost immediately after eating). It noted that there were many fine toothpastes and powders for sale, but also gave a recipe for one with precipitated chalk, oris root, and oil of peppermint, suggesting dentists' continued distrust of commercial products. The pamphlet told children to chew their food well to strengthen their teeth. Finally, it suggested two visits to the dentist a year – on one's birthday and six months later. At the time, doctors too recommended a periodic health exam, with the birthday as a reminder.[81]

The Ontario Dental Association's longer and more scientific *Joy of Living*, for older children and parents, proposed preventive health as the way of the future: "No matter how clever or ambitious a person may be, it will be almost impossible for him to reach the top without good health." Good teeth would help to ensure first-rate health. *Joy of Living* emphasized taking care of baby and permanent teeth. It instructed parents to keep their children from using pacifiers or sucking their thumbs or mouth, which might cause permanent deformities. It also included lots of information about preventing "pyorrhoea" (gum disease) through good food, exercise and sunshine, regular bowel movements, and keeping the mouth clean and correcting any abnormalities in the mouth. In line with the theory of oral sepsis, it warned that pyorrhoea could lead to dire consequences including rheumatism, "now believed to be almost wholly an infectious disease," and tuberculosis, as well as listlessness and colds. It concluded with some dental axioms including "Many a man digs his grave with his teeth."[82]

In addition, the CDHC itself offered *At the Gate* (similar to *Treasure House*), and another pamphlet confusingly also called *Joy of Living*. It sponsored films, including *Tommy Tucker's Tooth* and *Bobby's Bad Molar*.[83] The CDHC's *Joy of Living* also stressed good oral hygiene for success in life. It emphasized prevention and urged students to strive for health and keep their teeth strong by exercising them frequently (by chewing hard foods) and brushing them regularly. For the BC campaign, the British Columbia Dental Association and the Canadian Dental Hygiene Council created *The Health Guards* (figure 1.1), a colourful pamphlet featuring a cabbage, apple, and celery stick mounted on horses made up of potatoes and carrots. They brandished toothbrushes as their swords.[84] *Guard Your Health*, distributed in Manitoba and Alberta, reminded readers that your teeth, if healthy, could be your friends, helping you to chew your food, and ensuring your mental and physical well-being. Neglecting them could make them "enemies," leading to stomach ulcers, digestive disorders, rheumatism, heart lesions, ear and eye trouble, bronchial problems, and nervous conditions – a reference to the theory of focal infection.[85] *The Health Guards* emphasized baby teeth and cautioned against mouth breathing, pacifiers, and thumb-sucking. It warned that poor oral hygiene would cause children to fail academically. The booklet taught people how to brush their teeth and recommended use of dental floss or tape, a balanced diet, thorough chewing of the food, and a visit to the dentist every six months. Another pamphlet, *Champions Keep Fit: Do You?*, for high schools, suggested that healthy mouths could improve athletic performance. It warned against cakes and sweets and promoted fresh fruits, eggs, vegetables, whole grains, milk, and vigorous chewing of food to exercise jaws.[86]

Walt Disney's black-and-white, silent film, *Tommy Tucker's Tooth* (1922), was a parable featuring friends Tommy Tucker and Jimmy Jones – Tommy developed proper health habits, while Jimmy became careless, thinking that brushing teeth was "only for girls." (Indeed, the limited evidence suggests that women brushed more frequently than men.)[87] Jimmy develops a terrible toothache, which prevents him from sleeping or studying. The film explains that food caught in the teeth would spoil and lead to an acid that would create a hole in the tooth. When the hole became deep enough to reach a nerve, the toothache would start. The film threatens that boys with toothaches might be

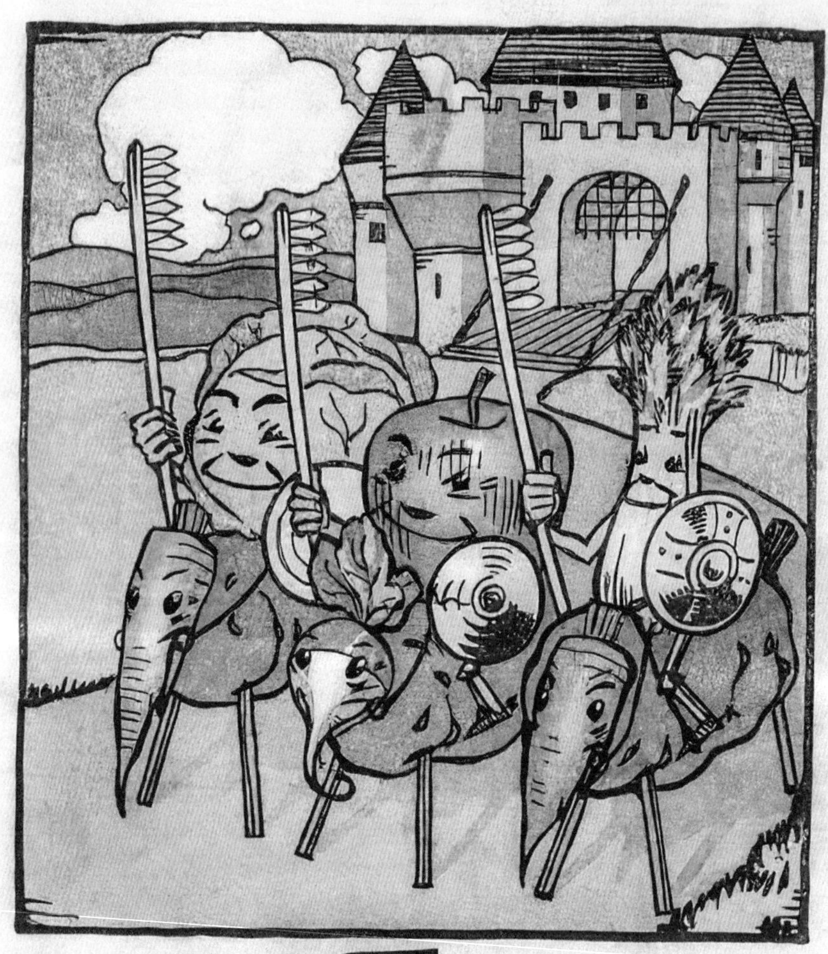

1.1 *Health Guards* pamphlet (1930) from the British Columbia Dental Association. More than 55,000 copies were circulated in 1930. The vegetable soldiers are brandishing toothbrushes as their swords.

underweight and undernourished. When the two friends look for a job, the chubby Tommy, with his toothy smile, finds work, while Jimmy, flashing his decayed teeth, is told that his lack of pride in himself suggests that he would not take pride in his work. The prospective employer counsels him: "Don't forget that the dentist is your best friend." Jimmy has his teeth fixed at the dentist, and the employer gives him another chance.[88]

Bobby's Bad Molar (1929) begins when Bobby develops a toothache and is sent to the school's dental hygienist. With a mirror, she shows him how food could stick in the crevices of the teeth and form an acid that would lead to cavities. His mother takes him to the dentist to have the tooth filled. At school, he is asked to explain to his classmates what he has learned, and he teaches them how to brush their teeth properly.[89]

Lessons about oral health continued to appear in schoolbooks as well. *The Ontario Public School Health Book* (1925) strongly recommends eating hard foods to keep the teeth sound, massage the gums, and develop the shape of the face. It suggested that brushing teeth twice a day was sufficient – morning and night – and recommended using camphorated chalk as a tooth powder. It proposed visiting the dentist at least once per year.[90] In 1926, Ontario introduced its first Dental Health Day and arranged for instruction on mouth care throughout the province.[91] As well, radio shows about oral health were broadcast for five nights in Toronto. Although the rest of the province did not receive five nights, there were broadcasts in Bowmanville, Brantford, Hamilton, London, Prescott, and Preston. Teachers were provided with a dental guide, and schools sponsored essay contests and art competitions. There were posters, newspaper advertisements, stickers for automobiles, and window displays. Organizations and schools showed films and performed a dental play, "A Bad Baby Molar."[92]

Under the activist leadership of F.J. Conboy, whom we met above, Ontario's Division of Dental Services established school clinics, and he urged hospitals and factories to begin offering a dental service. He arranged for dentists to visit rural areas that lacked practitioners.[93] Teacher trainees received lectures on preventive dentistry,[94] and the CDHC followed suit in other provinces.[95] In the late 1920s and early 1930s, Conboy worked hard to offer dental inspections and dental care to northern Ontario.[96] In 1930, the province's Department of Health cooperated with its Department of Education to provide dental clinics on train cars that called at communities too small to have a school. Conboy reported that nearly 100 per cent of people took advantage of the care provided, indicating a huge need for dental treatment. He also helped set up a dental clinic at the sprawling, annual, late-summer

Canadian National Exhibition in Toronto – a number of companies donated supplies, and toothbrushes, toothpaste, and mouthwashes were given away to patients.[97] In the 1930s, the dental rail service was expanded to cover a variety of rail lines throughout Ontario.[98] In Saskatchewan, the Junior Red Cross equipped two motorcars that travelled to rural schools across the province.[99]

Beauty, Etiquette, and Dental Hygiene

Dentists and doctors were not the only source of advice about mouth hygiene. Some people may have decided to brush their teeth not for their health, but to become more popular or receive a job offer or a marriage proposal. A review of the leading nineteenth-century etiquette and advice manuals suggests that a clean mouth did not seem as important as a clean body. Lord Chesterfield's famous *Advice to his Son, on Men and Manners* (1799) esteemed a clean mouth but offered no instruction.[100] *A Young Woman's Guide* (1846), by physician, educational reformer, and prolific writer William A. Alcott (a second cousin of the author Louisa May Alcott's father), recommended daily bathing but said nothing about brushing the teeth or caring for the mouth. He suggested mastication to exercise the teeth.[101] His guide for young men condemned chewing tobacco despite its reported merits as a tooth cleanser, and warned that licentiousness would lead to tooth decay in addition to a wide array of other ailments, but gave no instructions for brushing the teeth, despite a brief chapter on bathing and cleanliness.[102] *The American Code of Manners* (1880) called for good breath for gentlemen and suggested rinsing the mouth with cologne and water but, again, said nothing about brushing teeth.[103] By contrast, *The Bazar Book of Decorum* (1870), which focused far more on beauty than other guidebooks of the period, recommended that children brush their teeth or rinse their mouths after every meal. Adults should remove particles of food with toothpicks and brush teeth regularly with a little soap. The book advised against regular cleanings by the dentist, "who ought not to be allowed to file and scrape the teeth merely for the purpose of giving them an artificial regularity and whiteness not bestowed by Nature."[104]

The twentieth century saw an explosion of advice guides, some of which, like the *Bazar Book of Decorum*, paid more attention to beauty. The most famous etiquette adviser, Emily Post, dwelt on manners and behaviour and said little about the importance of personal cleanliness. But Sophie Hadida's *Manners for Millions* (1932) insisted on a daily bath to avoid body odour ("B.O."). Parents should teach children how to brush their teeth and tongue to avoid bad breath: "Though a person is in fine physical condition, there often is noticeable another form of B.O. (breath odor) caused by a film which quickly forms on the teeth and the tongue of some persons even though they take good care to brush them at least twice a day." Those "afflicted" should use an antiseptic mouthwash frequently – all food odours were offensive, and people ought to avoid onions and garlic.[105] Gayelord Hauser's *Eat and Grow Beautiful* (1936) had chapters on skin, hair, teeth, eyes, and nails. Smiling was part of women's charm, Hauser insisted, but only if their teeth were "white, strong and healthy." He advised eating a diet high in calcium and vitamin D. Vitamin C would protect the gums, while daily brushing with tooth powder would prevent decay.[106]

Advertising Toothbrushes and Toothpaste

While many parents and children would have had some exposure to this oral hygiene education through newspapers, pamphlets, the classroom, films, and advice guides, it is likely that far more of them learned to brush their teeth through advertisements for toothbrushes and toothpastes. In the 1920s and 1930s, a thriving market for toothpastes emerged in North America, as part of the new trend towards mass marketing of consumer-care products, such as soap.[107] In the United States in the 1910s and 1920s, as Kathy Peiss has shown, the number of perfume and cosmetic manufacturers nearly doubled and the factory value of their products increased by tenfold.[108] Canadian women spent far less on cosmetics than their sisters across the border, but their expenditures were rising.[109] According to advertising historian Vincent Vinikas, US toothpaste advertising increased thirtyfold between 1914 and 1931.[110] A "cupboard survey" of American homes in 1938 found that 64.6 per cent reported having toothpaste and 69 per cent at least one toothbrush.[111] By the 1930s, toothpastes were said to be one of the most competitive items in the pharmaceutical trade.[112] In this section, I examine Canadian toothbrush and toothpaste advertising by sampling oral hygiene ads across the country in *Chatelaine*, *Eaton's Catalogue*, *Revue moderne*, the *Saskatoon Star Phoenix*, Toronto's *Globe*, and the *Toronto Star*.

Toothbrushes as we know them today first came into use in China more than 500 years ago. By the nineteenth century, they were widely available in North America. Until the invention of nylon bristles in 1938, they were usually made of hog bristles. Handles were made of bone.[113] In the late 1930s, natural bristles gave way to nylon, and plastic began to replace ornate bone and metallic handles.[114] Toothbrushes were widely available in Canada soon after 1900, although it is unclear how often they were used. An article in *Maclean's* in 1910 suggested that fewer than 8 per cent of Americans used a toothbrush.[115] American dental researcher Joseph Kauffman estimated that in 1929 only 30 million toothbrushes were purchased in his country every year, for a population of 120 million. As bristle toothbrushes needed replacing every 3–6 months, regular brushing was apparently unusual.[116] In a later article, Kauffman reiterated, "There is good reason to believe that not more than 20 per cent of the population use a toothbrush."[117] This may be too pessimistic: in 1924 the American Child Health Association surveyed 35,000 schoolchildren: 68 per cent reported brushing their teeth "yesterday," perhaps reflecting expected norms more than actual practices.[118] A *Maclean's* article in 1932 indicated that fewer than a million toothbrushes were sold in Canada that year, similar to previous years: "This looks as if the average Canadian buys a toothbrush once in twelve years, say five in a lifetime. What it actually means of course, is that a large part of the population doesn't use toothbrushes at all – which no doubt accounts for the fact that very few dentists are laying up their motor cars or appearing in breadlines."[119] But a 1950 survey of Ontario schoolchildren aged 5–15 found that over 90 per cent of both urban and rural children reported having a toothbrush. This suggests an enormous shift in less than two decades; it may reflect increased prosperity after the war, declining toothbrush prices when nylon bristles were introduced, and changes in people's toothbrushing habits.[120] Or it may indicate that families shared toothbrushes and replaced them less frequently than experts advised.

A wide range of companies were producing toothbrushes, and department stores and pharmacies regularly listed them for sale among a range of items.[121] Johnson & Johnson promised that its Tek toothbrush (introduced 1928) was better shaped than its competitors and had better bristles.[122] Dr. West's Tooth Brush was smaller and "scientifically shaped," and its advertisements showed how to brush teeth properly.[123] The HI-GEN-IC toothbrush claimed to fit comfortably in the mouth, with bristles carefully placed to penetrate between the teeth and reach the back of the teeth.[124] Boxes holding Pro-phy-lac-tic toothbrushes touted that "A Clean Tooth Never Decays." The box suggested brushing twice a day and visiting the dentist four times a year.[125] In the 1930s, the same product promised that its rounded bristles were superior to competitors'.[126] Sanitol reported that "Dentists Recommend" its tooth and toilet preparations, including toothbrushes.[127]

The far bigger market was for toothpaste, and for every toothbrush advertisement, there were dozens for toothpaste. In 1932, Canadians reportedly spent $1,598,349 on toothpaste, or roughly one tube per person every 18 months.[128] Ads for this product, like those for soap, promised beauty, romance, and success.[129] They also stressed the marvels of science. Ads for Pepsodent, a leading brand, promised to "remove the film on teeth" and make them "glisten." Many featured attractive young women looking in the mirror (figure 1.2).[130] As Jane Nicholas has shown in *The Modern Girl*, personal appearance was becoming increasingly crucial to young women, whose social lives and employment often depended on their appearance.[131] Pepsodent's ads claimed that "modern research" underlay its toothpaste and often offered a free 10-day tube to consumers who wrote to the company.[132] They invoked the wonders of "science," implied the approval of the dental profession (some featured a young woman together with her dentist), and promised beauty.[133] In the 1930s, Pepsodent also began appealing to mothers, warning that "backwardness in school of a great many children is caused by neglected teeth" while avowing that its toothpaste was gentle enough even for baby teeth.[134]

In the mid-1930s, Pepsodent began claiming that both its toothpaste and its tooth powder contained Irium – a "thrilling new discovery" that "out-performs anything in dentifrice history for restoring luster!"[135] Its ads did not describe this miraculous new ingredient in any detail – it was actually a combination of different sulphated alcohols shown to clean better than soap.[136] But the single word "Irium" bestowed scientific authority and perhaps generated less stigma than "sulphated alcohol" in an era when some people still supported temperance and prohibition. Many commentators associate ingredient branding with the "Intel Inside" computer campaign of the 1980s, but clearly it has been around for much longer.[137] Putting Irium in tooth powder, a product bouncing back thanks to Depression-era nostalgia for earlier, simpler times, combined the wonders of modern science with old-fashioned wisdom. Pepsodent was likely trying to compete with Dr. Lyon's tooth powder, which was taking off in the 1930s. In 1927, Lyon's was purchased by the R.L. Watkins Company, which invested heavily in advertising the product. These ads stressed that dentists used powder, which was cheaper than toothpastes because consumers were not paying for water.[138] Not surprisingly, attention to cost surfaced strongly in toothpaste marketing during the Depression.

In the 1940s, Pepsodent began running a series of advertisements featuring attractive female adult twins: one twin used Pepsodent tooth powder; the other did not, providing "laboratory proof that Pepsodent powder makes teeth 32% brighter than the next leading brand."[139] This campaign seems to have been copied from a Pebeco campaign that ran in the early 1930s,and purported to show that the twin who brushed her teeth with Pebeco had gleaming teeth, while,

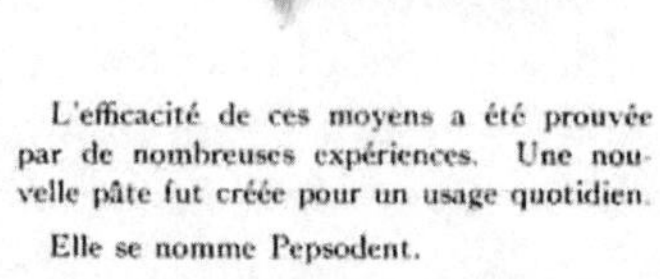

LA REVUE MODERNE 57

Pour Vous

Des dents plus blanches que des millions de personnes sont fières de montrer

Maintenant de quelque côté vous vous tourniez, vous voyez partout des dents plus blanches et plus saines.

Ceci est le résultat d'une nouvelle manière de se nettoyer les dents, employée par des millions de personnes. — Faites-en l'essai et constatez par vous-même le résultat.

Combattez la pellicule.

Les dents sont recouvertes par la pellicule — cette pellicule visqueuse que vous sentez. Bientôt cette pellicule se décolore et forme une couche malpropre. C'est pourquoi les dents deviennent noirâtres.

De plus la pellicule retient des substances qui fermentent et forment un acide. Elle maintient l'acide en contact avec les dents ce qui cause la carie. Des millions de microbes y naissent. Ces microbes avec le tartre, sont la principale cause de la pyorrhée.

Peu de personnes évitent les ennuis de la pellicule avec les anciennes méthodes de brosser les dents.

Les experts en dentisterie ont maintenant trouvés deux manières de combattre ces pellicules. L'une désagrège la pellicule, l'autre l'enlève sans frottement nuisible.

L'efficacité de ces moyens a été prouvée par de nombreuses expériences. Une nouvelle pâte fut créée pour un usage quotidien.

Elle se nomme Pepsodent.

Son usage s'est répandue dans le monde entier, grâce au conseil des dentistes.

Résultats Remarquables

Pepsodent augmente l'alcalinité de la salive ainsi que son pouvoir d'assimilation de l'amidon. Il donne à la nature un plus grand pouvoir protecteur. Les résultats combinés vous étonneront.

Envoyez le coupon pour un essai gratuit. Constatez comme vos dents sont propres après l'avoir employé. Remarquez l'absence de la pellicule visqueuse.

Voyez comme les dents deviennent plus blanches à mesure que les couches de pellicules disparaissent.

Vous serez toujours heureux de l'avoir essayé. Découpez ou copiez ce coupon immédiatement.

Protégez l'émail de vos dents.
Pepsodent désagrège la pellicule, puis l'enlève au moyen d'un agent plus mou que l'émail. N'employez jamais, une substance contenant des particules dures.

DE FABRICATION CANADIENNE

Canada

Pepsodent

Enrégistré

LE DENTIFRICE NOUVEAU

Basé sur des recherches scientifiques modernes. Conseillé par les principaux dentistes du monde entier.

Découpez ce coupon immédiatement.

1621 Can.

Tube de 10 jours, gratuit.

THE PEPSODENT COMPANY
Département 481, 191 rue George, Toronto, Can.
Veuillez expédier un Tube de Pepsodent de 10 jours à

....

....

(Un tube seulement par famille).

1.2 Like many toothpaste advertisements, this 1925 ad for Pepsodent shows a young woman examining herself in the mirror.

in the words of one critic of toothpaste advertising, "the other twin presented a sickly smile disclosing front teeth that looked as though she had just finished a portion of blueberry pie."[140]

Notably, Pepsodent also sponsored the most popular radio show in the United States, *Amos 'n' Andy*, a racist program that featured two white comedians portraying African-American migrants from the south, raising the ire of some Black Americans (and likely Black Canadians as well).[141] Canadian ads for the toothpaste often mentioned the show was available on the National Broadcasting Company (NBC) and included pictures of the two comedians in blackface (figure 1.3).[142] While it is not known if these cut-outs were used in Canada, Pepsodent provided US drugstores with racist cut-outs of "Amos 'n' Andy"– portrayed in character, with huge, lipsticked mouths – carrying giant tubes of toothpaste.[143] As Ben Medeiros argues, it is no coincidence that a toothpaste that promised "whiteness" became entangled with racist representations of blackness. Pepsodent was not alone in tying toothpaste to racist imagery – Darlie toothpaste, one of the most popular brands in Asia until Colgate pulled it off the shelves in 2020, was known as "Darkie" toothpaste from 1933 to 1989 and featured a white man in blackface on its packaging.[144]

While Pepsodent could remove "film" from teeth, Colgate averred that its "cleansing foam" could reach parts of the mouth competitors could not. It differentiated itself by attesting to its honesty in advertising. Unlike products that claimed to cure pyorrhoea and firm up the gums, it suggested that anyone with concerns about their teeth or gums visit a dentist.[145] It emphasized the care of children's teeth – its pamphlet *The Way to Happytown* told the adventures of Bob and Betty, included a toothbrushing chart, and offered a Health Club Pin for brushing teeth regularly.[146] Even so, some of its claims were hard to support. A 1931 ad featured endorsement from several scientists who claimed that Colgate's foam cleaned better because it reached into "tiny crevices in between the teeth" and removed decaying food. While lauding the product's scientific merits, it also termed its cleaning power "truly magical."[147] In 1934, the American Dental Association removed Colgate from its list of accepted products for false advertising.[148] In the 1930s, Colgate ran frequent ads boasting that it was cheaper and worked just as well as more expensive brands.[149] In 1935, it began a new campaign, one likely inspired by Listerine mouthwash's very successful "halitosis" commercials. Listerine's cartoon-format ads, ubiquitous in the 1920s and 1930s, featured attractive young women who could not figure out why their boyfriends had left them for someone else, or why they could not obtain a date, until a kindly friend suggested that they had

FREE . . . *a 10-day tube of Pepsodent*

Film
is found by dental research to discolor teeth and foster serious tooth disorders.

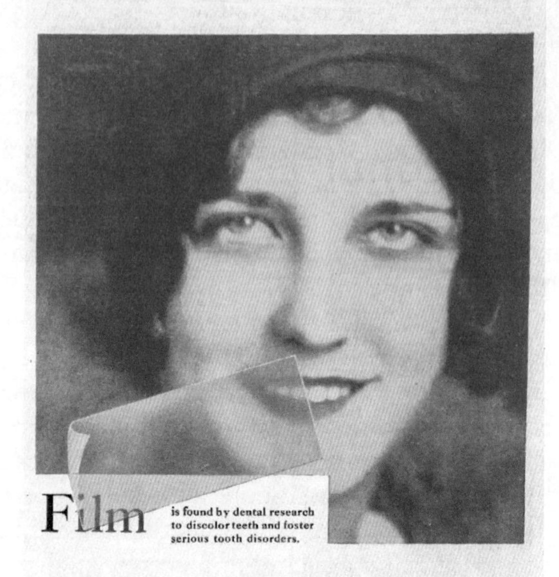

These Germs Incite Tooth Decay

Millions are imprisoned on your teeth by film

This special method that removes film and bacteria will be mailed you free to try. It may bring a great change also in your teeth's appearance.

THIS advertisement is published to ask you to accept and try a tooth paste entirely different from all others on the market.

By the time your free supply is gone these things will have happened to your teeth: *stains and discolorations will be gone—decay combated at the source—the incidence of many other troubles controlled.*

The great destroyers of teeth are highly active germs. Germs cause decay. Under favorable conditions they, with tartar, are a contributory cause of other troubles, too. Many ways are known to kill bacteria. *But on the teeth bacteria cannot be removed by ordinary methods.*

A sticky, stubborn film envelops them. It glues germs against the enamel and in the tiny cracks and crevices. There they multiply by millions. *To remove these germs you must remove germ-laden film.*

Pepsodent was developed after years of laboratory study and experiment. Pepsodent removes film gently, safely.

Pepsodent does not contain pumice, harmful grit or crude abrasive.

The Most Popular Radio Feature
AMOS 'n' ANDY

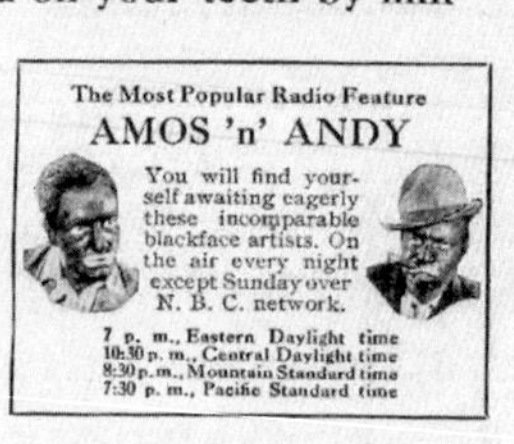

Please accept a supply to try

Pepsodent is not a "cure" for decay and pyorrhea. It is a preventive. The diseases, themselves, must be treated by your dentist. Tear out the coupon and send it to the nearest address . . . today.

Use Pepsodent twice a day. See your dentist at least twice a year.

FREE 10-DAY TUBE

Mail coupon to
The Pepsodent Co.,
Dept. 806. 191 George St.,
Toronto 2, Ont., Can.

Name ....
Address ....
City ....

Other Offices: The Pepsodent Co.,
919 N. Michigan Ave., Chicago, Ill., U. S. A. 8 India St., London, E. C. 3, Eng. (Australia) Ltd., 72 Wentworth Ave., Sydney, N.S.W.
Only one tube to a family 3459-Can.

Pepsodent
The Special Film-Removing Dentifrice

Pepsodent, the tooth paste featured in the Amos 'n' Andy Radio Program

1.3 Pepsodent promoted its sponsorship of the racist *Amos 'n' Andy* radio show in its Canadian advertisements, here in *Chatelaine* (June 1930).

halitosis. Listerine quickly solved the problem, and weddings ensued.[150] Colgate's version of what Roland Marchand has described as "shame" advertisements suggested taking a toothpick or some dental floss to clean between the teeth. If there were food deposits on the pick or floss, it suggested smelling them. Did they smell bad? If so, the ad revealed, your teeth were not properly cleaned. Colgate could correct the problem and clear up the bad breath.[151] One such cartoon suggested that "Joan" found a job once she banished her bad breath, thanks to Colgate. Now, she was living in Montreal – and out on a date as well![152] Similar romantic themes involved a Colgate-using high-school student getting a date, and a young wife whose husband has been neglecting her is taken out dancing by her spouse after she starts using Colgate.[153] In the late 1930s, Dr Allan Roy Dafoe and the world-famous Dionne Quintuplets, from Callander, Ontario, endorsed Colgate, leading to an ad campaign showing the "Quints" sliding down a tub of Colgate and frolicking with their toothbrushes (figure 1.4).[154] Dr Dafoe reportedly chose Colgate because children liked the flavor.

In the meantime, bad breath's threat to romance extended to men as well. In a 1944 ad, a young woman will not go to a dance with a young man because of his bad breath, while in 1945 a sailor loses his girlfriend for the same reason but wins her back after using Colgate.[155] The gender reversal would appear to reflect the changing dating and marriage market prompted by men's return home at war's end and the new emphasis that men were expected to place on home and family.[156]

Ipana toothpaste warned of the dangers of "pink toothbrush" – a supposed sign of gum disease. It highlighted the dangers of modernity, warning that "modern foods, so soft, so rich, threaten the health of your teeth and gums" and stressed the importance of exercising the gums through massaging them with a finger or toothbrush, using Ipana toothpaste.[157] The idea that "primitive people" had much better teeth was a truism in the dental literature of the day, which held that modern diets, including too much sugar, were ruining people's teeth. As Roland Marchand points out, the parable of "civilization redeemed" – the idea that modern life had disadvantages that could be overcome through the purchase of the advertised good – was one of the dominant themes of interwar advertising. One clever Ipana advertisement featured an elegant woman chewing on a bone: in the text, a beauty editor pronounced it as "appalling" while a dentist praised it as "admirable" (figure 1.5).[158] A series of Ipana ads in the late 1930s featured women who generally took care of their appearance but were "dental cripples" because they had ignored the warning signs of "pink toothbrush." The advertiser suggested a visit to the dentist, who would

30
CHATELAINE, APRIL, 1938
IT CLEANS OUR TEETH
AND MAKES THEM SHINE
PROTECTS OUR SMILES
JUST LOOK AT MINE
BESIDES ITS FLAVOUR'S VERY FINE!
ANNETTE
CECILE
EMILIE
MARIE
YVONNE
The Quins used Colgate's today.
Did you?
COLGATE
WHY DR. DAFOE CHOSE COLGATE'S DENTAL CREAM FOR THE DIONNE QUINS
Dr. Dafoe chose Colgate's Dental Cream for the little Dionnes because it cleans so *thoroughly*, yet so *gently*—without the slightest harm to delicate enamel . . . or irritation to tender gums.
And how the Quins *enjoy* brushing their teeth with Colgate's! Like all children, they love its delightful peppermint flavour — an important help in teaching correct habits of oral hygiene.
WHY YOU'LL LIKE COLGATE'S DENTAL CREAM, TOO . . .
Colgate's soft, safe polishing agent not only cleans enamel to shining smoothness . . . its special *penetrating* foam gets into those tiny hidden crevices between teeth that ordinary cleansing methods fail to reach . . . cleans every surface of every tooth . . . gives new brilliance to your smile . . . keeps your breath sweet and beyond reproach! Get a tube today!
LARGE SIZE 20c
GIANT DOUBLE SIZE 35c
MEDIUM SIZE 10c
COLGATE'S RIBBON DENTAL CREAM

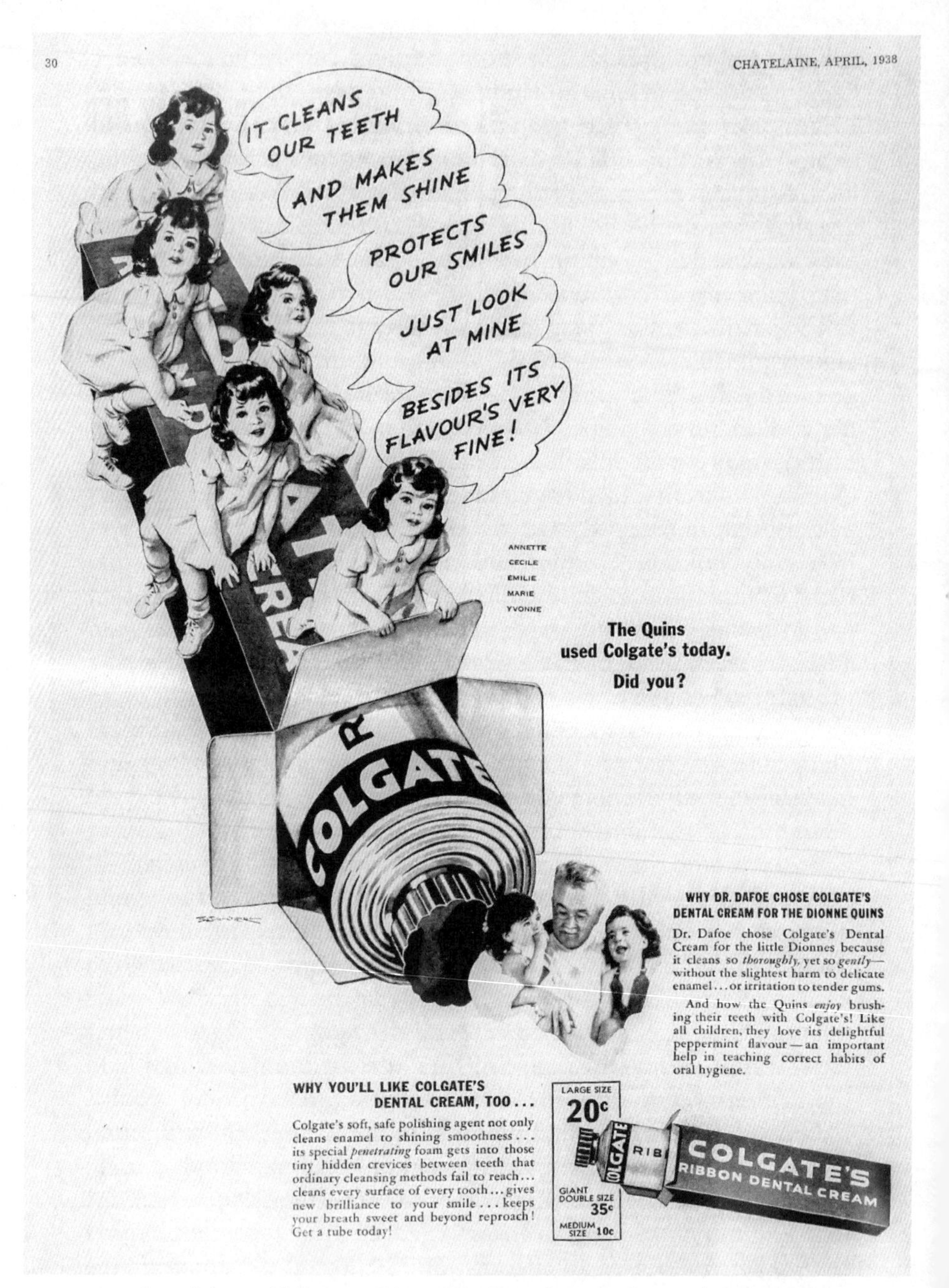

1.4 Canada's world-famous Dionne Quintuplets are shown sliding down a tube of toothpaste in this Colgate advertisement from 1938 in *Chatelaine*.

"APPALLING!" SAYS BEAUTY EDITOR
"ADMIRABLE!" SAYS YOUR OWN DENTIST

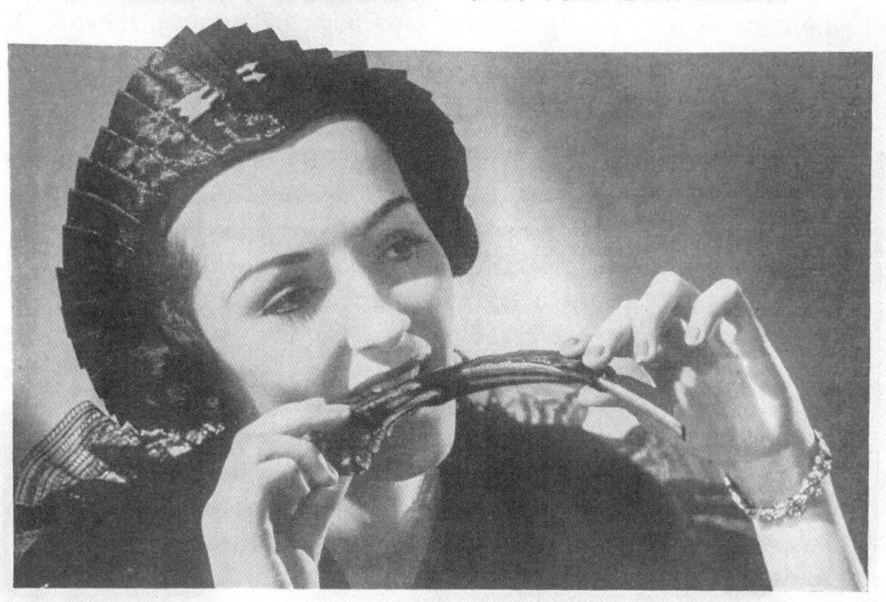

IT ISN'T BEING DONE, BUT IT'S *One Way* TO PREVENT "PINK TOOTH BRUSH"

"THAT'S a very shocking and unpleasant picture," says the Beauty Editor of a famous woman's magazine. "Any woman who behaved as badly as that would soon find most doors closed to her."

But your dentist would be equally emphatic—in quite another way.

"I'm for that picture," would be his prompt verdict. "I hope Ipana publishes it everywhere. For if people ate more rough, coarse foods—gave teeth and gums more work, more exercise—we dentists would not be forever warning them about the dangers of tender, sensitive gums—about 'pink tooth brush.'"

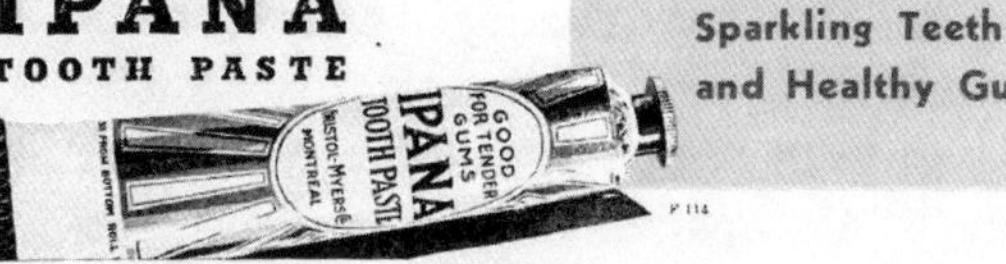

Of course, all dentists know that our modern soft-food diet does not give the gums that brisk, health-making work they need. They get lazy, tender . . . and some morning, the warning signal of "pink tooth brush" appears.

DON'T NEGLECT "PINK TOOTH BRUSH"

If you are wise you will begin today the *double* duty you must practice for complete oral health. For gums need massage as much as teeth need cleaning. So follow the teachings of modern dentists. Rub a little Ipana into your gums when you brush your teeth.

IPANA and Massage mean Sparkling Teeth and Healthy Gums

Ipana with massage helps stimulate circulation. It helps gums recover their health. And when gums are normal, you need have little fear of serious gum troubles—gingivitis, pyorrhea and Vincent's disease.

Start with Ipana and massage. For whiter teeth. For healthier gums. For a more attractive smile. And for protection against the troubles that may follow "pink tooth brush."

WHY WAIT FOR THE TRIAL TUBE?

Use the coupon below, if you like. But a trial tube can be, at best, only an introduction. Why not buy a full-size tube of Ipana today and get a full month of scientific dental care and a quick start toward firmer and brighter teeth.

• • •

BRISTOL-MYERS COMPANY OF CANADA, LTD.,
1239 Benoit St., Montreal, P.Q. CH-5-35
Kindly send me a trial tube of IPANA TOOTH PASTE free.

Name ____________

Street ____________

City ____________ Prov. ____________

1.5 In *Chatelaine* (October 1935) Ipana capitalized on the belief that so-called primitive people had better teeth. Other ads in the series featured women chomping on celery stalks, lamb chops, and carrots.

probably recommend more work for the gums as well as "Ipana and gum massage" (the latter elements conveniently being cheaper than the dentist).[159] Like Colgate and Pepsodent, Ipana often promised both career and romantic success.[160] Near the end of the war, its new series of humorous commercials featured cartoonish-looking women who were apparently unwilling to give up soft foods such as stew, pastry, and waffles.[161]

Squibb's Dental Cream warned people about "the danger line" where the gums met the teeth and acids could destroy teeth and gums. It promised that its special "Milk of Magnesium" could relieve "sensitive teeth" and soothe "sore gums" and was safe for both children and adults. Squibb, like many other toothpastes of the time, was invoking focal infection: "Thousands, dentists tell us, are stricken with serious illness – rheumatism – heart and nervous disorders – simply because of decaying teeth and infected gums."[162] Forhan's toothpaste claimed to cure pyorrhoea. It aimed for an older audience: a 1932 ad in *Maclean's* had a white-haired, well-dressed man in his mahogany-lined office, smoking a cigar. It warned: "Your dentist is wonderfully skillful … but the most beautifully made denture can never fully replace one's natural teeth, nor overcome the blow to one's self respect that follows their loss."[163] Another ad featured a tastefully dressed woman looking glum over a luxurious desk with a grand fireplace in the background. It said, "Many people really feel a keen humiliation when they lose a tooth." This ad suggested that children also use Forhan's, as it is "never too early for serious thought about teeth."[164] This brand stressed the importance of visits to the dentist twice a year.

Taken as a whole, this advertising proposed that everyone, both young and old, rich and poor, men and women, needed to brush their teeth regularly and that the benefits would go beyond keeping one's teeth. Good oral hygiene would improve one's job prospects, allow one to meet or keep a mate, improve one's health, and make one's teeth "glisten." While this advertising undoubtedly encouraged daily brushing of teeth, it appalled dentists, who were concerned about its inaccuracies. Before the introduction of fluoridated toothpastes in the 1950s, there was no evidence that any brand of toothpaste had any beneficial effect beyond freshening the breath, and perhaps encouraging brushing. The advantages of toothbrushing lay entirely with the act of brushing. In 1929, the American Dental Association formed the Council on Dental Therapeutics to research the claims of commercial dental products, which many dentists felt were false and misleading. To gain acceptance of their product as a "dental remedy," manufacturers needed to provide a full list of ingredients, and advertise their products truthfully.[165]

The opposition to false toothpaste advertising was part of a larger consumer movement that argued that ignorant consumers needed to be protected from unscrupulous manufacturers and advertisers.[166] Arthur Kallett and F.J. Schlink's *100,000,000 Guinea Pigs: Dangers in Everyday Foods, Drugs, and Cosmetics* (1933), one of the decade's best-selling books, included an entire section on toothpastes, excoriating Pebeco because its principle ingredient was poisonous, Pepsodent because it contained an abrasive that could damage tooth enamel, and Kolynos because it contained too much soap. It declared that "probably no other commodity has been responsible for so much downright and expensive lying by the respectable advertising agencies."[167] Schlink and Stuart Chase's *Your Money's Worth* (1936) lambasted toothbrush advertising as well, saying that no toothbrush could conform to the dental arch, that most in the market were too large, and that bristles tended to buckle and did not penetrate between the teeth.[168] In 1935, dentist Bissell Palmer, who had helped create the American Dental Association's Council on Dental Therapeutics, published *Paying through the Teeth*, a scathing account of the claims of toothpaste manufacturers. He worried that brands promising to cure "pink toothbrush" or clean between the crevices misled consumers into believing that they could care for their teeth properly without dental visits. Even so, most consumers likely knew little about the false claims of toothpaste manufacturers and purchased their products in search of a brighter smile.

Interwar education on dental hygiene by dental organizations, public-health officials, and advertisers appears to have made a difference. A 1955 study of the oral hygiene of Ontario civil servants found that people's dental hygiene declined as they aged. Only 36.9 per cent of civil servants aged 25–29 were found to have poor oral hygiene, compared to 68.2 per cent of those 50–54.[169] This might suggest declining attention to teeth as people aged, but around the turn of the century, when the older cohort was born, there was far less emphasis on daily toothbrushing, and its members probably did not take up the habit later in life.

Ironically, as Canadians began to brush their teeth regularly, some dentists began to question the practice. Dentists had always believed that diet helped prevent tooth decay, and interwar developments in nutrition intensified that focus. As food historians have shown, research in nutrition exploded in the 1920s and 1930s and many new vitamins were identified, revealing poor diet as the cause of many diseases, including dental caries.[170] In dentistry, the work of May Mellanby on vitamins D and A was particularly influential.[171] Some dentists, such as Weston Price, who was doing research on diets and dentition around the world, began to question the value of brushing altogether.[172] Russell

Bunting, a prominent dental researcher at the University of Michigan, blamed refined sugars for most tooth decay and proposed that mouth cleanliness, "except when carried to an extreme and impractical degree," did not provide "much protection."[173] William Brady, a physician who wrote a syndicated column on nutrition that appeared in many Canadian newspapers, also had doubts about brushing. Although very few dentists questioned the habit's merits, they started to acknowledge that "a surgically clean tooth is an impossibility in the normal mouth."[174] Or, as one Canadian dentist put it, "We no longer believe the old fallacy, 'a clean tooth never decays.'"[175] While public-health dentists never rescinded their advice to brush teeth, they acknowledged that tooth decay was more complicated than "mouth hygiene." The search for new solutions would bring them to fluoride and usher in a whole new era in dentistry.

2

Fluoridating Smiles

Transforming Oral Health

One of the best-known television advertisements of the late 1950s and early 1960s had children eagerly running to tell their mothers: "Look, Ma, No cavities."[1] The family was using Crest toothpaste with fluoristan. The announcer promised that it could reduce cavities by up to 50 per cent for the whole family. In 1960, Crest was the first toothpaste to be recognized as a cavity-fighter by the American Dental Association's Council on Dental Therapeutics. Two years later, it had more than 30 per cent market share.[2] The Canadian Dental Association (CDA) offered Crest similar recognition in 1971. Other fluoridated toothpastes followed, and by the end of the twentieth century, these products dominated the market in both countries. They probably helped facilitate the dramatic decline in dental caries in both fluoridated and unfluoridated communities after 1950. But they were not all that was on offer with regard to fluorides (which are ionized forms of the element fluorine). Water fluoridation became a hotly contested political issue, debated fiercely in many communities on both sides of the border. While the prevalence of fluoridated water is now declining, by the 1970s a little over a third of Canadians were consuming it regularly.[3]

As well, many children began receiving fluoride treatments at their dentist's office. At first, this meant painstaking application of fluoride to each tooth, but eventually fluoride gels, foams, and, most recently, fluoride varnishes simplified this process. School-based fluoride-rinse programs became common in the 1970s. Thanks in part to fluorides, by the late 1970s, many children had never heard a dental drill buzz, and some observers were predicting the end of tooth decay, although this proved to be overly optimistic.[4] Other factors besides fluorides helped reduce rates of tooth decay: better diet, childhood antibiotics, ongoing oral health education, and better access to oral health care. This chapter discusses fluoride interventions as well as the intensified campaign for oral hygiene between 1945 and 2010.

The Early History of Water Fluoridation

In the 1920s, advocates of "mouth hygiene" had hoped that regular toothbrushing would stem the ravages of tooth decay, but by the 1930s it was clear that this would not be enough. Even the cleanest mouths suffered from tooth decay.[5] Fortunately, for dentists determined to improve oral health, there was another solution on the horizon: water fluoridation. Its history begins at the turn of the twentieth century, when Dr Fred McKay, a Pennsylvania-trained dentist, moved to Colorado Springs, Colorado, to start a practice. Many of his patients had ugly brown stains on their teeth. Local people blamed the town's water, but he could find nothing about this in the dental literature. He began a wide correspondence to search for causes and eventually discovered that the so-called Colorado stain occurred throughout the Rocky Mountains, as well as in Texas, and in Italy and Portugal. But there did not appear to be anything unusual about the water in these places.

Then, in the early 1930s, a number of researchers, more or less simultaneously, discovered that the stain was caused by fluoride. Margaret Smith, a biochemist at the University of Arizona, created mottled teeth in rats by feeding them fluoridated water.[6] At about the same time, H.V. Churchill, the chief chemist for ALCOA (the Aluminum Company of America), discovered that the water in Bauxite, Arkansas, where residents had experienced mottled teeth since its water supply had been changed in 1909, had a high level of fluoride.[7] Fred McKay arranged for other places with a high degree of mottling to send sample water to Churchill for testing. All the water tested high in fluoride.

At first, fluoride was seen as a problem disfiguring teeth and rendering them brittle and difficult to repair. In the 1930s, Dr Trendley Dean, a dentist with the US Public Health Service (USPHS), began a widespread study of fluoride and tooth mottling (now called "dental fluorosis"). The USPHS wanted to determine what minimum level of fluoride in water damaged teeth.[8] It hoped that communities with too much could reduce the level of it or switch their supply. A number of researchers, including Margaret Smith and her husband, H.V. Smith, began working on filters to remove fluorine from water.[9]

But Trendley Dean made a crucial discovery: while high levels of fluoride were a problem, smaller amounts appeared to protect teeth. In 1938, he showed that children in places with 1 part per million (ppm) of fluoride in their water had less tooth decay than those in centres with none. At the end of his paper, he suggested that adding fluorides to the water supply might reduce tooth decay and called for more research.[10] Over the next few years, additional analysis revealed that cities with naturally fluoridated water had lower rates of cavities than those without.

By 1942, the USPHS was considering a study that would add fluorides to a city's water supply, but it needed to make sure that these would not cause any harm. First, would they have systemic effects on the human body? Clearly high levels of naturally occurring fluorides mottled human teeth – might adding fluorides affect the body in other ways? Fluoride accumulates in bone more than it does in teeth, so much of the research focused on bone health. Up to this point, the most extensive research on fluoride had been conducted by the Danish physician Kaj Roholm, on workers who handled cryolite, an unusual, fluoride-rich mineral used to make glass and aluminum. He found that most of these workers had osteosclerosis (harder, denser bones) and about one-fifth (20.5 per cent) had moderately or greatly reduced spinal mobility, such that some could no longer bend down to pick items up from the floor.[11] Some researchers worried about fluoride's effect on enzymes and on the thyroid.[12] There was also a history of crippling fluorosis in India.[13] Christopher Sellers has argued that the early fluoride researchers failed to take the Indian evidence seriously.[14] In fact, they did examine that research, but an extensive 1940 article on the subject noted severe famines and malnutrition as complicating factors, and the US researchers did not believe the situations comparable.[15] A 1941 paper in the *Journal of the American Medical Association* reported no sclerosis in communities with high levels of naturally occurring fluorides.[16] Within the USPHS, Frank McClure, the chief of the Laboratory of Biochemistry, began investigating the body's ability to excrete fluoride and how the substance accumulated in tissues, particularly skeletal. Other researchers, most notably Willard Machle and Harold Hodge, carried out similar investigations. They concluded that the body eliminated most of the fluoride and that there was no relationship between bone fractures and fluoride consumption. Most of the research, however, was done on younger men, so there was little sense of how fluoride might affect other groups. As McClure himself admitted: "Epidemiological studies of the non-dental effects of fluorine, as ingested in fluoride domestic waters, are extremely few in number and very limited in scope."[17]

Even so, many dental researchers were increasingly hopeful about the possibilities of water fluoridation and were keen to promote it. In 1945, the USPHS, the state of New York, and the city of Brantford, Ontario (soon to be assisted by the Canadian Department of National Health and Welfare), began studies of controlled fluoridation. While some people still expressed concern about the potential side effects, seven years of research had not produced any definite evidence of harm. The mid-twentieth century has often been regarded as the "golden age" of American medicine: infant mortality had plummeted, life expectancy had increased, new vaccines had significantly reduced infectious disease, and new drugs promised to combat bacterial infections.[18] Hopeful about what science and medicine could accomplish, some dentists and public-health officials used the beginning of controlled trials to launch a more concerted campaign for fluoridation. Fluoridation historian Donald McNeil has outlined the crusade led by Dr John G. Firsch, a dentist from Madison, Wisconsin, who provided his children with fluoridated water that he mixed at home and kept in his fridge. He labelled the tap water in his home as "poison." Together with Francis Bull, dental health officer at the State Board of Health, he campaigned for fluoridating water across the country, but especially in Wisconsin, where by 1950 more than fifty communities had adopted the measure. Firsch was a dentist, not a researcher, and he had little patience for the USPHS's detailed, careful studies. When several biochemists at the University of Wisconsin objected to the fluoridation of Madison's water supply in 1947, proposing fluoride tablets instead, Firsch claimed that they "didn't know a fluorosed tooth from a bed pan." Indeed, as both Ruth Roy Harris and McNeil argue, scientists at the USPHS were reluctant to endorse water fluoridation in 1950 but were ultimately overwhelmed by pressure from states' dental directors.[19]

Why were the latter so keen? First, the Second World War had highlighted the extent of dental disease in the United States and Canada. To join the American armed services, men had to have six opposing teeth in their upper and lower jaws; in 1941 this disqualified almost 10 per cent of recruits, and dental defects were the leading cause of rejection.[20] Dental leaders and public-health officials began to realize the extent of the need and began planning for more extensive dental care. In Canada, the wartime situation was similar: dental defects disqualified 23 per cent of enlistees.[21] After the war, preliminary studies by the federal department's Dental Health Division showed that more than 90 per cent of children over the age of eleven had tooth decay. By the time young people were fourteen, they had an average of twelve cavities in their permanent teeth. It would take a dentist six hours per child just to take care of existing needs. The CDA made it clear: there were not enough dentists to fill all those cavities. Reducing tooth decay was a must.[22]

As Alyssa Picard has shown, fluoridation related also to professional prestige.[23] Despite significant progress in dentistry between the wars, with better dental education and closer cooperation with doctors, practitioners still had a reputation as "merchants of pain" and worried about their professional prestige. In 1955, for example, Leroy Johnson, former dean of the Harvard School of Dental Medicine, proposed that practitioners, to increase their status, should serve more people, add more basic science to their education, cooperate with medical schools, and do more research.[24] Another dentist complained in the *Journal of the American Dental Association*: "A large segment of the public regards the dentist as he regards himself; namely, a repairman, nothing more. It never enters their minds that the dentist is a member of a learned profession." The dentist should, he insisted, emphasize prevention and "exert all his efforts toward solving the dental health problem."[25] In short, community water fluoridation was based on solid research and stressed prevention over cure: many believed it to be a panacea for dentistry's image problem.

Fluoridation also seemed like a boon to frustrated dentists who did not trust people to brush their teeth or eat less sugar. David Ast, director of New York state's Bureau of Dental Health and leader of the Newburgh–Kingston fluoridation experiment in the 1940s, noted two sure-fire ways to prevent tooth decay – eat less sugar and brush teeth after every meal – but they were "unrealistic," because "few people will adopt them conscientiously."[26] Dr Francis Bull, the state dental director in Wisconsin and a notable proponent of fluoridation, said that good oral hygiene, eating less sugar, and improving diet could reduce cavities, but he did not think the public was likely to do these things. Fluoride offered dentists the first real opportunity to prevent dental caries.[27]

By the early 1950s, the controlled studies were producing impressive results. After five years, cavities in Newburgh were down by 30 per cent, with even better results among the six-year-olds who had drunk fluoridated water for most of their lives.[28] In Brantford, Ontario, cavities among five-year-olds were down by 47 per cent.[29] There was reason to be enthusiastic, but not everyone was convinced. In 1950, Rep. James Delaney (D – NY) set up a House select committee to investigate the use of chemicals in foods and cosmetics, including water fluoridation. The full text of these hearings was published in 1952 and would provide considerable fodder for opponents of fluoridation. The committee heard testimony from public scientists, including Bruce Forsyth (assistant surgeon general and chief dental officer, USPHS), Trendley Dean (National Institute of Health), and John Knutson (USPHS). Forsyth explained that fluoridation had been more thoroughly studied than any other public-health measure and that it reduced cavities by two-thirds. Knutson and Dean described in detail the studies by the National Institute of Dental Research. When they realized the committee's scepticism about their findings, they also provided a bibliography of 64 references on fluoridation's safety and effectiveness, as well as copies of USPHS research papers.[30]

The committee also invited several opponents of water fluoridation. The first was Robert S. Harris, a nutritionist at the Massachusetts Institute of Technology (MIT), who did research on diet and dental caries. He was convinced that phosphate and other minerals could improve oral health.[31] He introduced a metaphor many anti-fluoride activists latched onto: If you have a headache and take aspirin and the headache goes away, that does not mean that an aspirin deficiency caused the headache. The fact that fluoride reduced cavities did not mean that humans required fluorides. Instead, he argued, we should be investigating the cause of dental decay.[32] He was also concerned about the long-term effects of fluoride consumption. Another opponent was Alfred Taylor, a biochemist at the University of Texas, who found that rats fed fluoridated water died earlier than the rats who were not. He had not yet published these results, and the USPHS, which had visited his lab to investigate the issue, believed them flawed.[33]

Researchers Margaret and H.V. Smith also testified against water fluoridation. She had been the first to determine that rats drinking fluoridated water could develop mottled teeth. She stated that fluorine did diminish tooth decay, but that even small amounts could mottle teeth, with notable psychological consequences. She pointed out that people, especially children, drink variable amounts of water, making it difficult to control the dose. Topical application of fluoride, she suggested, held greater promise, as did better nutrition and teeth cleaning. H.V. Smith also argued that use of fluoride, even at 1 ppm, would mottle teeth of many children. The Smiths lived in Arizona, where, as we saw above, several communities had high levels of naturally occurring fluorides in their water supply, and where heat increased water consumption, thus producing greater mottling even at recommended levels of fluoride. Indeed, USPHS scientists proposed adjusting amounts of fluoride for climatic conditions. Margaret Smith also worried about how fluoride might affect people with inadequate kidney function, and about the variable amounts of fluoride among foods, which complicated calculations of dosage.[34] In 1952, in short, there were still highly respected scientists expressing concern about fluoridation.

By 1954, when the House's commerce committee held more hearings on fluoridation, sceptical scientists from the Delaney hearings either were not invited or chose not to appear. In 1954, H.V. Smith publicly retracted his opposition after visiting Newburgh, New York, and stated that the mottling in Arizona had to do with climatic differences.[35] While doctors and dentists testified against fluoridation, they lacked the prestige of the 1952 experts. Leading the anti-fluoridation crusade in 1954 was a Seattle radiologist, Frederick Exner. Exner had been president of the local Antituberculosis League and of the State Radiological Society, but he had no record as a researcher. He complained that the leading fluoridation scientists were all just quoting and citing one another. He pointed to errors in Frank McClure's USPHS study of fluoride excretion, noted that children consume widely varying amounts of water, suggested that mottling was more severe than Trendley Dean's studies indicated, and pointed out that dentists found widely differing numbers of cavities. He condemned fluoridation as "totalitarian medicine" and described the trials at Newburgh and at Grand Rapids, Michigan, as a "flagrant violation of the most sacred laws of God and man."[36] While a number of Exner's concerns resembled those aired at the 1952 hearings, his passionate opposition to fluoridation, his attacks on the honesty and professionalism of fluoride scientists, and his scattered use of evidence devalued his testimony.

Dr George Waldbott, an allergist from Detroit, sent a statement. Waldbott, like Exner, was a respected physician–vice-president of the American College of Allergists – and had published more than 100 papers, mostly case studies.[37] He feared that 1 ppm of fluoride might not be safe for everyone, especially people with allergies or impaired kidney function. He worried that mottled teeth would not remain healthy over the long term and pointed out the challenge of tracing fluoride poisoning, since many of its symptoms (joint pain, malaise) were vague and could result from any number of conditions. He asserted that the best dental journals refused to publish anything opposing fluoride and that the American Medical Association had rushed its endorsement through its House of Delegates. His allegation of nefarious practices by fluoridation advocates (a consistent aspect of the opposition's discourse ever since) also irritated many dentists and research scientists who believed that researchers like Dean, McClure, and Hodge were investigating a legitimate scientific question in a fair, even-handed way. Meanwhile, a long-term study of two Texas towns – Bartlett (which had roughly 8 ppm fluoride in its water) and Cameron (about 0.4 ppm) – had eased concerns about fluoride's potential long-term effects on the body. In 1943 and 1953, researchers conducted medical histories, physical and dental exams, and blood and urine analysis on long-term residents of both communities and found no significant differences in their health, except for a high rate of dental fluorosis in Bartlett.[38]

In the years to come, Exner and Waldbott would become the leading scientific anti-fluoridation voices in both the United States and Canada. In 1957 they published *The American Fluoridation Experiment* with a mainstream press. James Rorty, a left-wing journalist with a longstanding interest in food and pollution, edited the book.[39] In clear, passionate prose, the authors termed the fluoride experiment an unprecedented expansion of the powers of public-health officials vis-à-vis citizens' lives; said that it would medicate entire communities for the benefit of only a few; and called for more research about fluorides, which would accumulate in the body, damage bones, teeth, and joints, and cause gastric distress. The best way to reduce cavities, they maintained, was to cut sugar consumption, and they asserted that the Sugar Research Foundation was a leading force behind fluoride promotion. In the chapter "Big Brother Knows Best: Budding Authoritarianism in Our Public Health Service," Exner argued that bureaucrats sought to expand their authority, while the aluminum and fertilizer companies that produced fluoride wanted more profits.[40] In 1955, Waldbott and his wife started the tabloid-style *National Fluoridation News*, which became crucial reading for anyone opposing fluoridation. The newspaper featured conspiratorial headlines, shocking revelations of pro-fluoridation tactics, scathing denunciations of fluoride's dangers, and funny cartoons.

As communities across the United States and Canada debated adding fluorides to the water supply in the 1950s and 1960s, proponents regularly stated that there was no legitimate opposition to the project and that dentists, doctors, and scientists were unanimous in their approval. This was not true. There were opponents in these fields, but, as the debate grew more heated, and the scientific evidence mounted in favour of fluoridation, the experts who had initially expressed hesitation either changed their minds or absented themselves from the debate, leaving the opposition largely in the hands of a few crusaders. The extreme views expressed on both sides created a hostile atmosphere for researchers who opposed the idea. Eventually, sceptics established their own journal, *Fluoride*, which published only articles critical of fluoridation.[41] Most scientists doing research in the field were very clearly identified as pro- or anti-, which confused the public. Whom should people believe? The reassuring pamphlets that labelled fluoridation safe, effective, thoroughly tested, and endorsed by experts? Or the opponents' far more lengthy and detailed books, leaflets, and pamphlets, which prophesied joint problems, heart and kidney disease, and cancer? That scientists and doctors appeared so divided may have made many people suspect that the experts were hiding evidence of possible harm. As the most thorough review of debates on fluoridation showed, the public felt it was being asked to decide on the safety of fluoridation during referendums and thus often chose caution.[42]

Fluoridation Referendums

Canadians voted consistently against fluoridation when they were asked in local referendums. Two of Canada's largest cities, Vancouver and Montreal, never fluoridated their water supplies. In Canada, as across the border, a range of groups lobbied for fluoridation, especially Home and School Associations and the Junior Chamber of Commerce. On the national stage, the Health League of Canada, a health promotion body led by Dr Gordon Bates, was the most notable promoter. In its magazine, *Health*, the League charted the progress of fluoridation, rebutted the most common criticisms, and blamed anti-fluoridationists for manipulating evidence, harming children, and impeding progress. Opponents tended to run their campaigns out of health-food stores. While they relied heavily on the work of the Americans Exner and Waldbott, several, less-prominent Canadian physicians supported them. In 1969 in the *Canadian Doctor*, an editorial from a Dr K.A. Baird condemned fluoridation's harm to enzymes and claimed that it increased the incidence of "mongolism" in children, tumour growth in mice, and bone disease in adults. Indicative of the anti-fluoridationists' sometimes-unsavoury political associations, the Canadian League of Rights, a racist group opposing fluoridation, circulated Baird's editorial to its members.[43]

Across the country, provincial and municipal laws varied widely on how a community could implement water fluoridation. In Nova Scotia, Manitoba, and Saskatchewan, it was up to the municipality to decide whether or not to do so. In Ontario, the choice was the municipality's, unless 10 per cent of electors petitioned for a referendum. In New Brunswick and Alberta, municipalities were required to hold a plebiscite before acting. Initially, Alberta required a two-thirds majority for the referendum to pass; in 1966 this was reduced to half of voters. British Columbia required a local referendum to approve of fluoridation, with 60 per cent to pass. Newfoundland and Prince Edward Island had no legislation on the matter; nor did Quebec until 1975, when its Liberal government mandated compulsory fluoridation throughout the province, although the ruling Parti Québécois suspended this legislation two years later. Some provinces also helped local authorities pay for equipment if they were fluoridating.[44]

Not surprisingly, supporters were keen to proceed without referendums. They believed that fluoridation was safe and effective and that it was a scientific matter beyond the competence of the general public. More importantly, they worried that having a referendum lent legitimacy to opponents and allowed scheming anti-fluoridationists to mislead the public. In 1962, CDA President Dr William Miller of Vancouver argued that fluoridation was a scientific decision and that "the idea of holding plebiscites to decide on fluoridation is a lot of nonsense – an insult to anybody's intelligence."[45] By contrast, many politicians saw the issue as a political hot potato and preferred to let the voters decide.

Both pro- and anti- forces spoke about the impact of fluoridation on health. Supporters announced that fluoride would improve general health by reducing tooth decay by as much as 65 per cent.[46] Opponents argued that fluoride caused heart disease, cancer, birth defects, kidney problems, and skeletal changes, and that some people were violently allergic to it. It is not surprising that water fluoridation, a measure that would benefit primarily children's health, was heavily promoted during the baby boom of the 1950s and early 1960s, when the health and well-being of children became a major focus.[47] Some opponents expressed resentment of this child-centric agenda. Some elderly people raged that while fluoride might improve children's teeth, it would endanger their health. One Calgarian asserted indignantly that "aged citizens are in no position to chance such a poison in their daily tea, coffee or soup."[48] Many opponents claimed that fluoride in the water would worsen their bladder or kidney problems.[49] This opposition among some Canadian seniors hints at the group's growing political consciousness (a trend traced by James Snell in *The Citizen's Wage*), as well as an intriguing dissent from the era's child-centred culture.[50]

As the debate continued, the antis emphasized the risk of cancer. In the 1970s, the US National Health Federation, which supported "freedom of choice" in medicine, employed anti-fluoride activist John Yiamouyiannis. At the time, the National Health Federation was a leading proponent of laetrile, the controversial anti-cancer treatment, and opposed vitamin regulation. (Its Canadian affiliate, the Consumer Health Organization, started in 1977.) Together with biochemist Dean Burk, Yiamouyiannis began publishing studies – not in peer-reviewed journals but as booklets – that purported to show that cancer death rates were much higher in fluoridated communities.[51] Leading scientists quickly pointed out that adjusting these figures for age and race removed the differences. Even so, the cancer claims received such wide publicity that health authorities in both countries investigated the putative link. Canada's Environmental Health Directorate found no statistically significant differences in death rates from any type of cancer in centres with and without fluoridated water. Nevertheless, antis kept raising the cancer scare, as well as a range of other health risks, as reasons for boycott.[52]

One of the opponents' strongest arguments was against involuntary consumption of a substance, even if it reduced tooth decay and caused no harm. Toronto's conservative-leaning *Globe and Mail* decried water fluoridation as "an infringement of personal freedom."[53] Jean Drapeau, the long-time mayor of Montreal (1954–57, 1960–86), who is often blamed for the city's lack of fluoridation to this day, used this argument. He believed that fluoridation would improve children's teeth, but he did not think that the state should force the issue, even if a majority passed a referendum.[54] Women's groups opposed to fluoridation often took a similar position. In 1976, for example, the Provincial Council of Women of British Columbia resolved that "the right to determine what shall be done to one's own body is fundamental and one should not be forced to take medication that has not been approved for that particular body."[55]

Anti-fluoridationists suggested that children – the people who needed it – could be given fluoride tablets, which ensured proper dosage. Supporters retorted that tablets were more expensive, that parents could hardly be expected to give their children tablets daily for more than a decade, and that having a large amount of fluoride in the home increased the risk of accidental poisoning. Antis countered that parents who could not administer fluoride tablets were simply lazy.[56] Thus fluoridation entered the vast debate over what constituted good parenting.

Both sides also invoked economic arguments. Supporters stressed reduced dental bills. A National Health and Welfare pamphlet from 1955 claimed that fluoridation would cost 10–17 cents per person per year – about the same as a loaf of bread.[57] In 1975, Quebec's minister of social affairs, Claude Forget, estimated only 10–12 cents per person per year and added that it would save taxpayers $40 million in school dental programs in just ten years.[58] By contrast, antis complained that most water was not drunk, but used for washing, watering lawns, and so on, and therefore it would be more cost-effective for individuals to add fluoride to their own drinking water. Typical was a 1971 letter from Saskatchewan: "99% of the water goes needlessly down the drain ... This is foolishly expensive."[59] In fact, in large urban centres with economies of scale, fluoridation was an inexpensive public-health measure. But objecting to the cost of fluoridation allowed some taxpayers to express their view that dental costs should be assumed by the individual, hinting at a more general opposition to the welfare state and its perceived threat to individual liberties.

Fluoridation debates took place at the height of the Cold War, and, given the conservative politics of many anti-fluoridationists, some resorted to conspiracy theories to explain why so many seemingly respectable persons favoured fluoridation. In Stanley Kubrick's ironic 1964 cult classic, *Dr. Strangelove*, General Ripper launches an all-out nuclear attack against the Soviet Union, explaining that the communists were destroying "our precious bodily fluids." He described water fluoridation as "the most monstrously conceived and dangerous communist plot we have ever had to face."[60] While Kubrick's film mocked Ripper, arguments that fluoride would be used to make the population docile or would allow communists to poison the water supply were common in the 1950s in both the United States and Canada. In a tract widely circulated in Canada, W.B. Herrstrom, editor of the *Americanism Bulletin*, claimed that fluoride provided "a ready weapon for saboteurs" and that it "breaks down the 'wills' of the people."[61] In Vancouver, Rev. Herbert Robinson's pamphlet "Fluorides – the Poisoning of a Whole Race" blamed a communist plot.[62] As Gretchen Reilly has argued for the United States, the bulk of opponents eventually steered away from the communist-plot line, largely because it opened them to ridicule (like Dr Ripper in *Dr. Strangelove*).[63]

From the mid-1950s on, a common anti- argument was that fluoridation helped the aluminum industry, in particular ALCOA, to rid itself of a toxic waste product that was otherwise very expensive to dispose of properly. However, there is no evidence that ALCOA or other aluminum companies ever promoted water fluoridation or that they made much money from producing fluorides for water fluoridation.[64] In blaming "big business," opponents had much in common with populist movements, like Social Credit in western Canada, which blamed centralized bankers for the Depression, but also appealed to left-wingers concerned about growing corporate power and irresponsibility.[65]

One of the most frequent arguments from the 1950s through the 1970s was that putting fluoride in the water was not natural. One citizen interviewed by the *Toronto Star* retorted, "Yes, I don't think nature intended that we should put chemicals in the water. We should drink it as pure as it can be."[66] Vancouverites regularly emphasized protecting Vancouver's "famous" and "exceptionally pure" water.[67] Drawing on a widespread anti-modernist sentiment, some antis contended that dental decay was a disease of "civilization" and that eating more natural foods would obviate the need for fluoridation. Dr W.J. McCormick wrote: "Let us study the eating habits of primitive men. In contrast to 'civilized' people, primitive men had splendid teeth, perfectly formed dental arches, sound bones, and well-formed bodies."[68] It was only when people started eating "devitalized foods" that tooth decay set in. Some anti-fluoridationists said that people should cut back on soft drinks, sugar, and refined foods. Reflecting their preference for private rather than public solutions to health problems, they felt that the real issue was "permissive" parents. One mother wrote that she was "one of the 'ignorant' who opposes fluoridation and must be looked after for my own good." She reported that her dentist had commented on her children's fine teeth and boasted: "Our children have soft drinks only for celebrating occasions, and candy as we buy it, not as they buy it. The moral, of course, is for parents to have some control over their children."[69]

Opponents also argued that, even if fluoride did occur in nature, the type being added to water (sodium fluoride or hydrofluosilicic acid) was not the same as that in nature (calcium fluoride).[70] To counter this, doctors and dentists began to turn the "nature argument" around. In 1978, the CDA's brochure "Nature's way to fight tooth decay" emphasized that fluoride is found naturally in "nearly all streams and other ground water," but that nature "doesn't always add just the right amount."[71] But, as the environmental movement gathered steam in the early 1970s, it became increasingly difficult to argue for adding another chemical to the water supply.

In the 1970s, opponents increasingly emphasized the pollution threat and danger to aquatic life. In 1967, airborne fluoride pollution from a fertilizer plant in Dunnville, Ontario, damaged crops and animals. Several residents claimed they were also suffering from fluorosis. This very real disaster provided opponents with ammunition. Dr K.A. Baird warned that fluoridating water could do to people what happened to animals around Dunnville.[72] In the early 1970s, the Pure Food Guild of British Columbia circulated a brief: "Our entire ecology is already suffering pitifully from pesticides, additives, drugs and pollution of all types in air, land and sea! Why add even more by polluting out water with a poison that is 15 times more powerful than arsenic?"[73] Miro Kwasnica, an NDP legislator in Saskatchewan, also cited environmental grounds. He warned the legislature: "Fluoridation of water supplies is nothing more than *legalized pollution* [*sic*] of our streams, rivers, lakes and oceans. I abhor it, as I do the use of insecticides, pesticides, sprays, food additives, white bread, white sugar and pop."[74] As the debate heated up in Quebec in the late 1960s, environmental groups, such as the Society to Overcome Pollution (STOP), became key players in the opposition to fluoride. In 1971, STOP published a lengthy research report by nutritionist Carol Spindell Farkas, which argued that, while fluoridation reduced cavities in children, it would add another chemical to "our already polluted water system."[75]

The idea that fluorides were accumulating, and that people were possibly approaching an unsafe dose, was spreading in the 1970s. This, of course, had much in common with the growing alarm over the fallout from nuclear testing. In the early 1960s, researchers and activists showed that the radioactive isotope strontium-90 was accumulating in children's teeth.[76] In 1963, Jean Marier, Dyson Rose, and Marcel Boulet, researchers at Canada's National Research Council (NRC), writing in the *Archives of Environmental Health*, called for research on possible fluoride accumulation and its impact on health. In 1971, and again in 1977, Marier and Rose, in their NRC report *Environmental Fluoride*, noted that fluorides were increasing in air, food, and water, so that residents of fluoridated communities were approaching dangerous levels of consumption.[77]

In response, the CDA sponsored a critical review of Marier and Rose's work. Jack Hann stated that their estimates of total fluoride intake were approximately double that of other researchers. He advised that the World Health Organization's monograph on fluoride consumption provided a much fairer review of the possible hazards. In 1979, the Canadian Public Health Association concluded that fluoride consumption was well within safe limits. None the less, from the 1960s on, Marier and Rose's research would attract widespread attention and be repeated in anti-fluoridation material on both sides of the border, most notably in the well-respected American journal *Saturday Review*.[78]

In the decades after 1945, Canadians across the country expressed strong unease about water fluoridation. While doctors and dentists were overwhelmingly in favour, opponents raised the alarm. Insisting that the issue needed more study, they predicted health problems such as cancer, kidney disease, and birth defects; suggested more effective, less wasteful ways to get fluoride into children; argued that fluoridation denied individuals' right to choose; and insisted that it was not natural. By the 1970s, the communist-plot theory (never that prominent) had largely disappeared, and the opponents latched onto the dangers of environmental pollution and cancer. But in most respects, they were remarkably consistent. From the 1950s through the 1970s, they expressed suspicion of large organizations, including the main medical and dental associations, as well as big corporations, and feared that the science behind fluoridation might be biased. Unlike the doctors and dentists who believed that only trained individuals could properly interpret and understand the science behind fluoridation, they were confident in their ability to critique the science and to do research, even if what they meant by research was often very different from that practised by professional researchers. In short, they opposed the technocratic ideals that Christopher Dummitt has shown were so crucial to the modernist project in postwar Canada.[79]

Anti-fluoridationists achieved considerable success. Although referendums passed in major Canadian cities like Toronto (by 50.7 per cent in 1962), Ottawa (62 per cent in 1964), and Edmonton (61 per cent in 1966), they were relatively narrow victories.[80] In both Ottawa and Edmonton, referendums had previously failed. In Vancouver, fluoridation failed three times, and in Calgary, four times before passage in 1999, removal in 2011, and passage in 2021. Quebec, as we saw above, ultimately suspended legislation mandating municipal fluoridation. By the 1970s, fluoridationists had lost momentum, and the number of fluoridating communities began to decline, as it still does.[81] Instead, dentists focused more on other ways of getting fluoride to children.

Alternatives to Water Fluoridation

Most dental researchers supported water fluoridation because adding fluoride to water closely emulated what occurred in nature. Perhaps because many of them had long been suspicious of commercial toothpaste (see chapter 1), they were slow to embrace fluoridated toothpastes in the 1950s. Moreover, initial studies of fluoridated toothpastes suggested that they were ineffective, although researchers eventually concluded that this was because the fluoride reacted with other ingredients in the toothpaste. In the first successful trial, in the early 1950s, a stannous-fluoride paste reduced decayed, missing, and filled surfaces by 72 per cent over six months.[82] A year later, the study was showing a 50.6 per cent decline in caries.[83] The same team then compared a sodium-fluoride toothpaste, a stannous-fluoride paste, and a control group. The children receiving the first saw statistically insignificant reductions in tooth decay, but those using the second had 45 per cent less caries after six months and 36 per cent less after twelve.[84] Together, these studies convinced dental researchers that fluoridated toothpastes were effective.

As we saw at the chapter's start, the first fluoridated toothpaste to become commercially available was Crest, launched in 1956. Crest came in a simple, medicinal-looking tube, implying it was for health, not vanity. Its advertising stressed that scientific studies had shown how it reduced tooth decay. According to toothpaste historian Peter Miskell, this therapeutic slant marked a major shift in toothpaste advertising, which had previously stressed cosmetic benefits.[85] A number of other toothpaste manufacturers quickly followed suit, including Brisk fluoride and Super Amm-i-dent.[86] In 1960, the American Dental Association's Council on Dental Therapeutics endorsed Crest. In response, manufacturer Procter and Gamble launched a new marketing campaign, heralding the endorsement and thanking the American Dental Association for its "public service." It had already advertised Crest heavily, but the imprimatur, along with the new advertising, catapulted the brand to number one. Crest cemented its early lead by advertising in the *Journal of the American Dental Association*, urging dentists to recommend Crest. Procter and Gamble also provided educational materials to schools, enclosing red tablets that children could chew after brushing – the red residue showed remaining plaque.[87] Many children, including me, loved seeing their stained teeth and learned how to brush better.

Ipana quickly jumped on the bandwagon, adding sodium fluoride to its toothpaste in 1961.[88] In 1964, the American Dental Association recognized Cue toothpaste (from Colgate-Palmolive, which had produced the best-selling Colgate before Crest came on the market).[89] But in 1968, Colgate-Palmolive replaced Cue, launching "Colgate with MFP" (sodium mono-fluorophosphate) with a major advertising budget, hoping to knock Crest out of top spot.[90] The new brand also had the American Dental Association's endorsement, but it failed to catch up to Crest.[91]

Advertisements for fluoridated toothpastes in Canada were aimed at a white audience. At that time, Canadian advertising rarely featured people of colour other than in racist or stereotypical ways.[92] Even still, the absence was glaring. A Crest ad of 1978 in *Chatelaine* featured photos of thirteen families, all of whom allegedly used Crest. Every family was white.[93] It was not until 1986 that a toothpaste advertisement in *Chatelaine* included a visible minority – Colgate featured an Asian child.[94] Crest followed suit in 1987 with an ad presenting multiple polaroid photos – one featured an adult Asian woman.[95]

By the mid-1970s, researchers were estimating that fluoridated toothpastes could reduce tooth decay by 28–32 per cent.[96] By 1981, 75 per cent of US toothpaste sold contained fluoride,[97] and by the 1990s, more than 90 per cent of toothpaste sold there and in Canada had fluoride as an ingredient.[98] A 1996 survey of fifty-two international experts on the post-1970 decline of caries in Western countries credited fluoridated toothpaste above all, but rated water fluoridation very effective where implemented (primarily in the United States, Canada, Ireland, New Zealand, Australia, Chile, and Argentina).[99] Indeed, some researchers believe that fluoridated toothpastes are even more effective than shown by clinical trials, which last only two or three years.[100] Not all experts agree: research from Sweden suggests that improved oral hygiene, less consumption of sweets, and fluoride prevention programs in schools were probably more helpful.[101]

There were other ways to use fluoride. One was regular applications of sodium fluoride or stannous fluoride to children's teeth. Basil Bibby, the dean of the prestigious Tufts College Dental School and later director of the Eastman Dental Center, pioneered such treatments. He believed that fluoride helped largely by combining with enamel to increase its resistance to acid. Unlike most researchers at the time, he believed that the effects of fluoride were topical, not systemic. In 1944, he reported reducing cavities by over a third in two years by applying fluoride solutions to adolescents' teeth.[102] Since the teeth needed to be thoroughly dried before application, and the fluorides needed to be applied regularly, this method was time-consuming and costly.[103] Bibby also tried to develop fluoride toothpastes.[104] In the 1950s, the "Knutson technique" of applying fluoride significantly reduced cavities, but took several days, tasted unpleasant, and stained the teeth.[105] In the early 1960s, fluoride gels could be placed in impression trays, which simplified the procedure.[106] Some had flavours like cherry or grape, which appealed to young patients.[107] Fluoride varnishes were introduced in the late 1960s in Europe. The hope was to increase the caries-reducing properties of fluoride by keeping it on tooth surfaces for longer than was possible with other fluoride products like foams and gels. These varnishes were slower to go into use in Canada but were widespread by the early twenty-first century.[108] They appear to reduce decay on permanent teeth and are easier to apply than fluoride gels and foams[109] and safer than gels, which can introduce too much fluoride.[110] In Canada, they are particularly recommended for high-risk children, although the teeth look yellow or dull for the 4–12 hours before the excess varnish is brushed off.[111]

Fluoride tablets or drops were another possibility, but their benefits had not been as thoroughly researched, and dentists worried about the chance of poisoning.[112] They were not as effective as community water fluoridation: more of the fluoride was excreted, and people tended not to take them consistently.[113] Another option that was rejected in Canada was fluoridated salt. Switzerland, which already had a long tradition of iodized salt, initiated the use of fluoridated salt in 1955. Fluoridated salt seems to have reduced cavities substantially, though in tandem with fluoridated toothpastes, so effects are hard to disentangle. Fluoridated salt is widely used in Germany as well.[114]

Fluoride rinses were first used in Scandinavia. In the mid-1960s, an extensive study in Sweden showed caries reduced by up to 50 per cent with daily rinses.[115] A promising US study in 1971 showed reductions of over 40 per cent. As a result, the National Institute of Dental Research sponsored seventeen community demonstration programs, which showed that significant caries reductions could be achieved with little cost. By the early 1980s, as many as 12 million children were participating in weekly programs.[116] But by mid-decade, randomized trials were challenging the rinses' effectiveness. It seems that the continuing decline in dental caries probably exaggerated their impact in the absence of controls. At a time when children were having fewer and fewer cavities, fluoride-rinse programs became less cost-effective and most appropriate for high-risk populations.[117]

The enthusiasm for such efforts had an impact in Canada. On Vancouver Island, a program was implemented in 1971 after a failed referendum on water fluoridation. It was a weekly rinse, coordinated by a "fluoride lady" and supervised by teachers and volunteers. Children were given napkins, a small paper cup containing the rinse, and a larger cup to spit the liquid into after swishing it through their mouths. By 1976, there were noteworthy declines in decayed, missing, and filled teeth among 13-year-olds. Their oral hygiene also improved – partly, the researchers believed, because the rinse program had helped valorize oral health.[118] Similarly, in Labrador in 1978, public-health nurses began a fluoride-rinse program in fifty-four communities that received only sporadic visits by a dentist.[119] In 1981, roughly 182,000 children in Ontario were rinsing with fluoride at school.[120] But these programs collapsed when spending on public dental health decreased in the 1980s.

Many children develop cavities on the pit and fissure surfaces of their first and second molars. In the 1960s, dentists began "sealing" these surfaces to prevent tooth decay. While the first-generation sealants often failed, new materials keep sealants in place for much longer. Some sealants contain fluoride, although its benefit is unclear.[121] In Saskatchewan, where until 1987 dental care was free for all children, that care included sealants.[122] They seem particularly effective in children prone to cavities.[123]

Educated Smiles: Oral Hygiene Education Expands

While fluorides spurred the decrease in cavities, oral hygiene also improved thanks to an explosion of oral health education after 1945, as all levels of government began to spend massively on public health, part of a larger expansion of health-care spending. Ottawa established a Dental Division at National Health and Welfare in 1945, and within a year it was focusing on children's preventive dentistry. In addition to producing educational material, it gave grants that allowed provinces, county health units, or municipalities to set up dental treatment for children often in remote regions where the need was greatest.[124] Over the next decade, most provincial departments of health established a dental division, many of which produced educational materials for teachers or hired dental hygienists to give presentations in schools.[125] Ottawa and the CDA also produced pamphlets. Quebec's Collège des chirurgiens-dentistes created a Ligue d'hygiène dentaire in 1939 to educate people through radio, newspapers, and demonstrations.[126] The Health League of Canada added a "Dental Health Day" to its National Health Week, while several provincial dental associations sponsored Dental Health Weeks.[127]

The Dental Division in Ottawa circulated pamphlets on oral health for mothers and included instruction on the subject in its educational materials for them. A frequently circulated item was *Your Baby's Teeth*, from the Dental Public Health Committee of the Ontario Dental Association. It told the story of Helen and Bess. Helen's doctor advises her to go see a dentist on learning that she's pregnant. "What's the matter with your teeth?" her husband asks. Helen responds:

> Not very much – although I never did have really first-class teeth. But the doctor says that the dentist's care, when you're going to have a baby, is very important. There is an old wives' tale that when you have a baby you have to lose at least one tooth – I've heard that dozens of times. It's nonsense. Maybe it used to be true, for good reasons – that is, the mother has to provide material to make her baby's teeth before it is born – that's what Dr. Hislop told me – and nature is very careful of that baby; it gets first choice. So the doctor tells women to add calcium and other bone-building material to her diet, not only so that the baby's bones and teeth will have enough material, but so that her own teeth will be well nourished and protected during her pregnancy too; and then the dentist watches them all the way along and makes sure nothing is happening to them. There's a gum condition called gingivitis that can occur in pregnancy, that really means sore and tender gums. The dentist can care for that too.

Self-deprecatingly (and in keeping with norms that urged women not to appear brighter than their husbands), she adds: "There, that's practically a lecture! I feel terribly learned." She says that she'll do everything the doctor tells her to, because "I want the nicest and prettiest and healthiest baby in the world."[128]

At her next visit, the dentist reassures her that if she takes care during her pregnancy, her child will not "inherit" her bad teeth. Her teeth decay easily because her early diet was not as good as it should have been. The pamphlet emphasizes that eating well during pregnancy will help to ensure strong baby teeth and permanent teeth for the child. Also, baby teeth must be healthy so that they fall out at the right time and leave the right space for their replacements.[129] The pamphlet included a menu for the mother to follow with lots of whole-wheat bread, fruit, vegetables, and milk – all highly recommended by nutritionists. When he was born, Helen's baby barely cried, and at six months he sprouted his first tooth with little fuss. His baby teeth grew in white, sound, and well-formed.

Helen's neighbour, the pamphlet tells us, is also pregnant. Bess is pretty but worn out from all the socializing that she and her husband do. She doesn't think that it is necessary to visit the doctor or a dentist while she's pregnant – after all, her mother had ten children, and it all worked out fine – those professionals are only for emergencies. Bess's baby slept poorly and kept the family up all night. When her teeth erupted, she lost weight, couldn't sleep, and was clearly miserable. They grew in crooked and discoloured – devastating for Bess, who, reflecting the gender ideologies of the day, said that if "a little girl isn't pretty, it's just terrible." The pamphlet concluded by admitting that it was exaggerating the impact of proper and improper care and urged mothers to consult their doctors and dentists.

National Health and Welfare also circulated the American Dental Association's booklet *Your Child's Teeth* (1940), a heavily illustrated, factual account of tooth development, which promoted breast feeding, advocated taking children to the dentist before the age of three to ensure a pleasant experience before the child needed treatment, warned against premature loss of baby teeth, advised brushing of teeth, cautioned parents about thumb-sucking and lip-biting, and recommended fresh fruit and vegetables.[130] A Canadian version was prepared by the Ontario Dental Association's Dental Public Health Committee in 1952 and circulated by both the Ontario and Canadian dental associations.[131] It emphasized that oral health was primarily a personal responsibility, and that children needed to be taught to brush regularly and avoid sweet foods and soft drinks. Like its American model, it stressed breast feeding, cautioned against mouth breathing and abnormal sucking, warned against the premature loss of baby teeth, and promoted the value of X-rays. It took a much stronger line against feeding youngsters candies, chocolate, jam, and soft drinks, explained how to brush teeth, and included Canada's Food Rules. The federal department's lengthy *Dental Health Manual* offered teachers much the same advice.[132] The department also inculcated oral health in its flagship publications on child and maternal health in English and French: *The Canadian Mother and Child* (which covered pre-natal care and the first year of life) and *Up the Years from One to Six*.

The National Film Board of Canada produced a number of films on oral health for the department. *Something to Chew On* (1948) emphasized the horror of becoming a "dental cripple." That term was common in the literature of the day, reflecting probably the new interest in "crippled children" brought about by mid-century polio epidemics as well as the era's ableism, and emphasizing how serious dental diseases were.[133] The film started with a pretty teenage girl, looking at herself in the mirror (reminiscent of interwar toothpaste ads). Sadly, her teeth are very damaged. The rest of the film focused on her family – her mother, Mrs Allan, was already a "dental cripple," her gums inflamed, and she had already lost several teeth. Will her children also become "dental cripples"? Not if they value dental care.

The film explained how teeth grow in the womb and during childhood and that they are essential for chewing food, aiding speech, and appearance – to illustrate the last, the film showed a man, likely in his fifties, without his teeth and then with his dentures. Like Ipana commercials, it stressed that the "mushy diet of modern civilization" failed to exercise the teeth enough. The film showed Inuit eating raw meat and asserted that because "this man lives on a rugged, primitive diet" his teeth were very good. It stressed a varied diet and underlined that many of the best foods were the cheapest. Pregnant women needed to take very good care of their teeth, and X-rays could reveal otherwise-invisible cavities. The film opined that "candy, gum and soft drinks are not so popular today" and reported that children liked to eat raw apples and carrots. Children should be taken to the dentist when they are three years of age – we see the youngest daughter, Ruth Allen, in the dental chair looking around at all the equipment while her mother waits outside. The film emphasized that many schools provided dental examinations as well: Jimmy Allen's card from the dentist showed that he had tooth decay and that he needed a space maintainer because some of his baby teeth had fallen out too soon.[134]

The animated feature *Teeth Are to Keep* (1949) was set in the Smith home, where baby "Junior" had just cut his first tooth. The film stressed the need for chewing to keep teeth healthy – just like the family dog chewed on bones, the Smiths kept their teeth healthy by eating raw

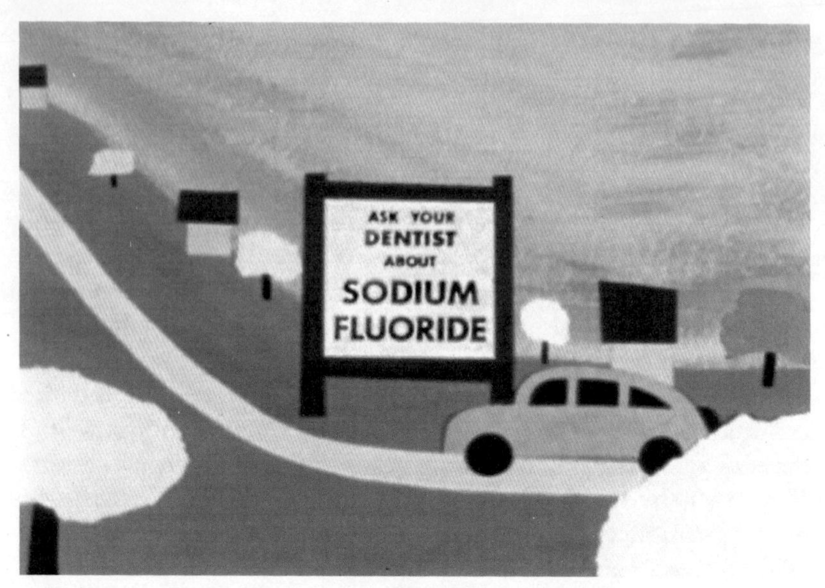

2.1 The NFB film *Teeth Are to Keep* (1949) featured an early plug for water fluoridation.

carrots, celery, apples, and salad. The father announced a picnic for the next day, and the eldest boy, Roger, was so excited that he almost forgot to brush his teeth after dinner. The film demonstrated what happens when a tooth decays and emphasized brushing immediately after every meal. Before the picnic, the Smiths checked that everything in the car was working – this was to emphasize that teeth, like cars, needed regular checks. They passed a sign saying, "Ask Your Dentist about Sodium Fluoride" (figure 2.1). After a delicious meal of brown bread, milk, tomatoes, radishes, apples, and meat, they rinsed their mouths with water – a substitute for brushing their teeth. In addition to promoting a healthy diet, the film encouraged children to see dentists as trusted health professionals.

There was a corresponding upsurge in oral health education in Canada's popular magazines, especially those geared towards mothers, such as *Chatelaine*, *Revue moderne*, and *Health* (often available in doctors and dentists' waiting rooms). This advice was very similar to Ottawa's, with a few exceptions. *Revue moderne* emphasized the role of good teeth in women's beauty, while *Chatelaine* frequently urged water fluoridation and applying fluorides to the teeth.[135] Both advised a well-balanced diet, recommended chewing hard foods to exercise the jaw, instructed people to brush their teeth four times a day, and were hopeful about what dentists could do for oral health.

In Quebec, the Ligue d'hygiène dentaire, which started in 1942, was extremely active. In 1959, for example, it made 554 radio and television broadcasts and circulated many news articles as well. It had eight full-time dentists on staff.[136] That year, the Ligue made 1½-hour presentations in all the schools of the Commission des Écoles Catholiques de Montréal. A representative of the city's Service de Santé spoke on nutrition, and the Ligue, on dental hygiene.[137] In the 1960s, the Ligue regularly showed *Gardons nos dents*, the French version of *Teeth Are to Keep*, described above. It offered a weekly column on dental hygiene in *La Presse* and other newspapers. The Ligue closed in 1965 as Quebec centralized health services during its Quiet Revolution – the five dentists on staff were absorbed by the provincial Division d'hygiène dentaire publique.[138]

In addition to a growing volume of educational materials, there were more school-based dental programs across Canada. Though often providing treatment, usually to lower-income children, they were primarily educational – teaching oral health to parents and children alike. The first such service began in Toronto in 1911. Dental public-health officers would visit schools and inspect children's teeth. Youngsters needing care received a card for their parents to take to a dentist, although one report said many parents found it difficult to locate any who were willing to treat children.[139] By the early 1920s, the program was employing three dentists. After a school inspection, the dentist spoke to the classes about oral hygiene. Montreal introduced its own program a few years later and by 1928 had three dentists on staff. By 1951, about two-thirds of schoolchildren were having their teeth inspected. Parents were encouraged to take their child to the family dentist if treatment was required; school clinics were only for children with "substandard" incomes. Clinics extracted teeth more often than filling them – in 1950, they extracted 28,661 and filled 9,671.[140]

By 1960, a review of Canada's dental public-health programs found that many provinces were employing dental hygienists for school inspections and education. In Nova Scotia's rural communities and small towns, for example, dental hygienists examined children's teeth, provided prophylaxis, offered instruction on brushing and diet, applied topical fluoride, and informed parents whose children needed additional treatment. In Quebec, 60 of the 74 health units offered dental services, which included education and dental inspection and, in some places, treatment to poorer children. Toronto continued to be a leader in the field. It employed 39 dental-health officers, a quarter of them full time. In 1959, 91 per cent of all Toronto children were examined. In Saskatchewan, approximately half of health units employed dental hygienists to apply fluoride topically and teach oral hygiene. Calgary, Edmonton, Vancouver, and Victoria also provided school inspections.[141]

The CDA strongly supported school inspections, which largely directed patients to the private dental office. In its brief to the Royal Commission on Health Services (Hall Commission) in 1962, it argued that "dental disease control is a matter of personal responsibility" and recommended properly cleaning the teeth, eating a balanced diet, and avoiding sweets. In its view, the best option for children's dental care was to universalize the school inspections that notified parents of treatment needs. Such programs, it maintained, could reduce dental disease by up to 50 per cent. It did not think that the state should cover restorative service.[142]

In the 1970s, oral hygiene education arrived on Canadian television with the *Toothbrush Family* (figure 2.2), an Australian animated series featuring child toothbrushes, Tina and Toby, their toothbrush parents, Tess and Tom, the electric toothbrush Hot Rod Harry, and Flash Fluoride (a toothpaste), as well as other common bathroom items. On these four-minute shorts, the toothbrushes came to life for adventure after the family had gone to bed. Most episodes featured the *Toothbrush Song* (with the melody of "Three Blind Mice") urging children: "Brush your teeth, round and round; Circles small, Gums and all." The goal of the series was to make toothbrushing fun.[143] The Ontario Ministry of Health produced a series of shorts featuring "Murphy the Molar" – one counselled against eating sticky foods, another emphasized wearing mouth guards for sports.[144] A Murphy the Molar mascot also made regular appearances at oral health education events and at schools in Toronto.[145] Other communities had their own version of "Murphy the Molar." In Penticton, British Columbia, "Toby Brush," a three-foot-high styrofoam toothbrush dressed as a cowboy dental-health sheriff, delivered a dental public-health program. The bad guy was "Sugar Bowl Pete," who had a face made of gum, cookies, pop, and cake.[146] Dental hygienists also became active educators. In Regina in 1973, the local branch of the Saskatchewan Dental Hygiene Association set up a booth in the local Woolco Department store for Dental Health Week. It showed films on various aspects of dental treatment and gave toothbrushing demonstrations.[147] Similar events took place across the country.

In the late 1970s, the CDA focused on Dental Health Month, partly because many dentists worried that denticare, discussed in chapter 3, might jeopardize their autonomy and professional freedom. A 1976 editorial in the *Journal of the Canadian Dental Association* complained that at the CDA's National Convention in St John's the previous year, the press kept complaining about Newfoundlanders' poor oral health,

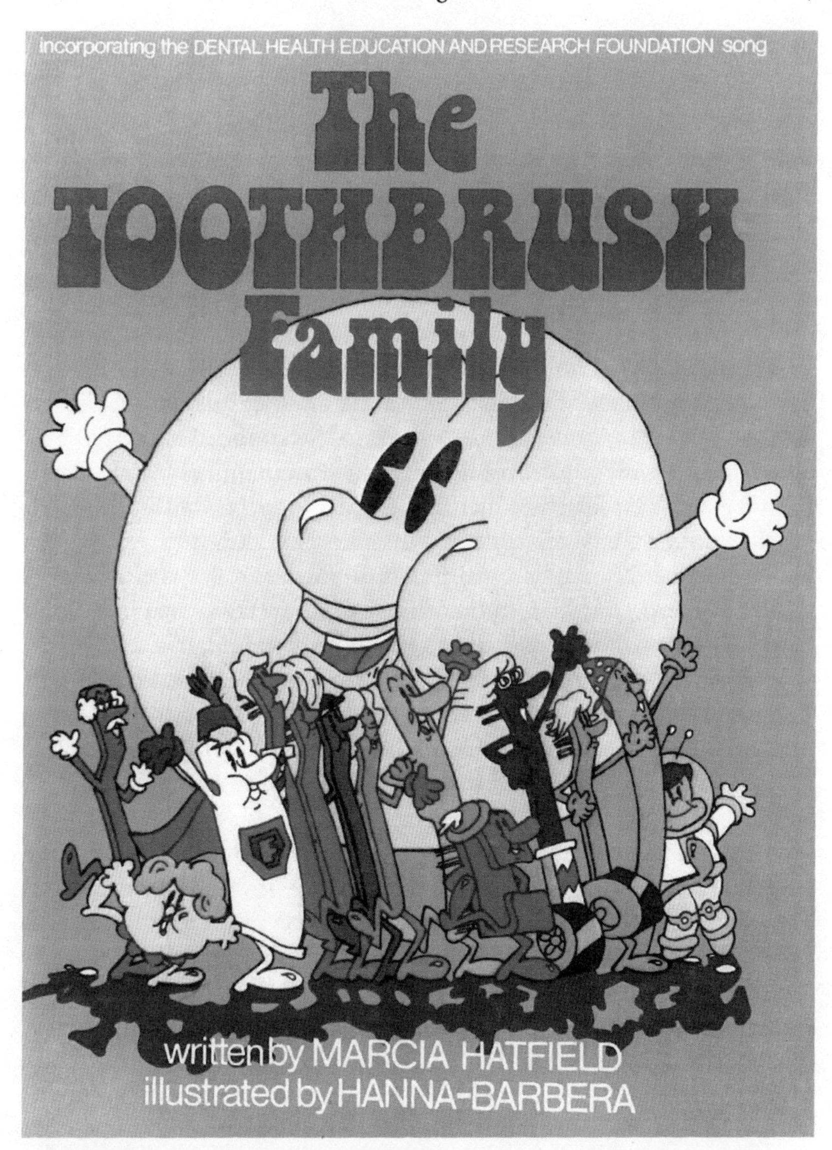

2.2 The book cover for Marcia Hatfield's *The Toothbrush Family* (1974). The animated Australian series of the same name appeared on Canadian television in the 1970s.

their lack of dentists, and costly dental care. The CDA's president, Fred Reid, reminded the press that "the tools for tooth brushing and flossing don't cost much and that dental health begins right in each person's mouth." The editorial argued that the press failed to report Reid's words and emphasized that "the public must be told and yes, sold, on the idea that all the money in the world won't buy them basic dental health. Dental health starts in front of their own wash basins with toothbrush, paste and floss in hand. It starts at their own table with the food they eat and the food on which they snack." It added: "If people continue to believe that their poor dental health is the result of dentistry's failure to provide dental care then the profession may well find government controlled dentistry on its doorstep, sooner rather than later."[148]

In 1980, the CDA hired the American ventriloquist Shari Lewis and her puppet Lambchop, well-known from the *Captain Kangaroo* TV show for children, to do commercials on oral health. It also hosted a nationwide poster contest, brush-ins, "Smile-a-thons," and dental displays.[149] One "Smile-a-thon" in Etobicoke (Toronto) had winners showing their upper front six teeth for over five hours.[150] In the mid-1980s, the CDA's Dental Awareness Program included Dental Health Month, a booklet, *The Consumer's Guide to Dental Care*, and other educational materials, many sponsored by Colgate-Palmolive. In the late 1980s, the campaign shifted away from health to promoting smiles, reflecting the profession's move towards cosmetic dentistry (traced in chapter 6). In 2007, Dental Health Month became Oral Health Month, recognition that oral health was about more than just the teeth.

Conclusion

When the Brantford fluoridation study started in 1944–45, the average 11-year-old in Ontario had 6.42 decayed, missing, or filled teeth;[151] 40 years later, the figure was only 1.26.[152] More and more children had never had a cavity. By the early 1980s, the decline in tooth decay in many Western countries had some observers speculating that dental caries was being eliminated.[153] The causes were multiple – community water fluoridation probably played a role, especially before the introduction of fluoridated toothpastes, although today the differences in tooth decay between communities with and without fluoridated water are small.[154] Fluoridated toothpastes, which now dominate the market, provided fluoride to ever greater numbers of people. A variety of other measures, such as fluoride-rinse programs in schools and fluoride gels and foams and dental sealants at dentists' offices, also helped. Childhood antibiotics and nutritional changes may have also played a role. In any case, this dramatic decline would have huge impact: it lessened the demand for publicly funded dental treatment, created a crisis among dentists who were not nearly as busy, and fed into the upswing in cosmetic dentistry.

3

Subsidizing Smiles

Public Dentistry for Designated Groups

In the late 1970s and early 1980s, dental care was simple for the Marchand family in Gravelbourg, Saskatchewan. The five children were treated at their school by a dental nurse / dental therapist who had been trained to do examinations, fill cavities, and clean teeth. After the province cancelled the Saskatchewan Health Dental Plan in 1987, obtaining dental care for the young Marchands became a lot more difficult. The family needed to travel 112 kilometres (70 miles) to Moose Jaw for every appointment. The mayor of Gravelbourg, as cited in the *Saskatoon Star Phoenix*, confirmed how the program's closure had hit his community: "At least our kids got their teeth seen to without missing a day of school. Now it costs time, gasoline, wear on vehicles and days off work."[1] The Marchands had benefitted from Canada's most successful children's dental program, in operation from 1974 to 1987. Its closure prompted mass protests and helped defeat the Conservative Devine government in 1991.[2]

In Toronto, Alan McPhee was not so fortunate. In 1970, he was an old-age pensioner receiving $114 a month when he had his remaining bottom teeth extracted. He had read that Metro Toronto would pay for a plate, but, unbeknownst to him, the relevant program was in arrears. When he went to apply for his plate, the nurse told him that his chances were minimal – the welfare office was prioritizing people who were looking for work. Without his bottom teeth, he could eat only soup, mushy foods, and bread that he soaked in liquid. He told the *Globe and Mail*, "I was always a meat eater … I really miss meat."[3]

Previous chapters have shown that brushing the teeth and fluorides both improved oral health, but dental treatment is also vital. In Canada, the provinces provide medical and hospital services to all citizens and permanent residents, but not dentistry. Today, public-health dentists complain that this country embodies the "inverse care law": people who need the most dental treatment actually receive the least, and vice versa.[4] The continuing socio-economic inequalities in the distribution of medical care are not nearly as severe as those in dental care. The national program of free physician care was introduced in 1968. By 1972, every province and territory provided free medical care to citizens, and most were considering offering free dental care as well.[5] Just as most doctors had opposed medicare, most dentists opposed the state provision of dental care, and health economists and health bureaucrats quickly concluded that it was too expensive, unless dental practice significantly changed. As a result, "denticare" never became a reality for most Canadians, except for children and recipients of social assistance in a number of provinces.

This chapter traces the debates over denticare and explores the history of state-funded dentistry in Canada. It does not include the services provided to Indigenous people, on whose inadequacy Ian Mosby and I have written elsewhere.[6] As Carlos Quiñonez has argued, uneven public funding reflects the widespread view that dental care is largely an individual responsibility, so governments pay for only people in special need (children, seniors, social-assistance recipients).[7] As Beatrix Hoffman has made clear, this is a form of rationing care.[8] While publicly funded oral health programs expanded in the years after the Second World War, growing notably in the 1970s, there were major cuts in the 1980s and 1990s.[9] The years since the mid-2000s have witnessed renewed attention to unequal dental care, a growing call for more public spending, and new investments aimed at targeted populations.[10] That said, there has been greater interest in pharmacare, which will probably win the race for public health dollars, as pharmaceuticals become more essential to our health.[11]

The Depression

During the 1930s, Canadians' enthusiasm for social programs, including public provision of healthcare, skyrocketed.[12] The Canadian Dental Association (CDA's) committee on state dentistry predicted some sort of "social health legislation" and urged dentists to think carefully about what it might look like.[13] In general, the CDA was very concerned about dentists becoming "servants of the state" and invoked the threat of "state dentistry" to drum up support for itself.[14] The American Dental Association's study of dentistry under compulsory health systems in Europe, excerpted in the *Journal of the Canadian Dental Association* (JCDA) in 1935, warned that the quality of service was poor. The American association's president reported: "The most vivid impression I have of dentistry in the European countries visited is a living, walking, glaring monument of false teeth. So far as I could learn, there is practically no program for public dental health education and little effort made to promote preventive methods."[15] Past President Dr Winter wrote that dentistry in US free clinics for the poor was much better.[16] A 1939 *JCDA* editorial complained that state dentistry would employ bureaucrats, but would not "provide adequate dental health for the nation." Instead, it proposed research into people's poor oral health.[17] Yet it did worry about accessibility. Another *JCDA* editorial acknowledged that treatment was too expensive for many people and that costs needed to come down – possibly through group practice and use of more auxiliary staff members.[18]

Nor was the profession unified. Some dentists during the 1930s expressed enthusiasm for state care, partly because their incomes were declining. Their US counterparts reported that average gross practice earnings fell from $4,000 a year in 1929 to less than $2,500 in 1935. Net incomes fell from $2,400 in 1929 to just over $1,000.[19] Similar data for Canada do not exist, but anecdotal evidence suggests that some dentists were suffering, especially in regions hard hit by the Depression. In 1935, one Saskatchewan practitioner described his increasing reliance on barter: patients with "abscessed teeth, swollen faces, pyorrhea, edentulous mouths, unbearable pain" were treated in return for beef, butter, ducks, fresh pork and sausage, geese, potatoes, a blacksmithing outfit, a cook-stove, fence posts, and hay, among other items.[20] Yet a survey by the Toronto Academy of Dentistry suggested that, at least in Toronto, dentists' incomes begin rising in the late 1930s. This may indicate that the recovery was starting even before the war, or it may reflect a flaw in the survey – apparently many dentists misunderstood the questions and answered them incorrectly. In the survey's "Comments" section, dentists were divided: some wanted public clinics closed to avoid competition, while others wanted more state care.[21]

In 1938, the Alberta Dental Association indicated its willingness to cooperate in "state dentistry," whatever that meant.[22] The *Calgary Herald* followed up and found that many practitioners worried that too few people received the dental care they needed. One reported recently fitting a denture for a woman whose teeth had been extracted fourteen years earlier, but she had been unable to afford a denture at the time. Now, her gums were so shrunken that she could probably never wear one. Another told of a patient who was having her teeth removed one or two at a time, even though she needed all of them extracted to cure her rheumatism. She did not think she would ever be able to afford dentures.[23]

During the Depression, there was some free care provided, especially for needy children. In many Canadian cities, local men's service clubs, including Rotary and Kiwanis, and women's groups organized such clinics.[24] In Quebec, the Junior Red Cross did the same.[25] Most large cities offered limited dental treatment to elementary-school students and to some welfare recipients. Provincial departments of health as well as voluntary health and welfare agencies provided some dental care in rural areas.[26] In the early 1930s, the Rosedale (Toronto) chapter of the Imperial Order Daughters of the Empire helped to fund a dental rail car that travelled across the province.[27]

In its 1938 brief to the Royal Commission on Dominion–Provincial Relations (Rowell–Sirois Commission), the CDA, rather condescendingly, posited four classes of people vis-à-vis dental care, revealing their condescension especially towards working-class patients. While the first class could afford dental care, "many of these people allow their teeth to decay and become a menace to their health." This group needed better education on how to care for teeth. The second class, which had mushroomed during the Depression, could afford only partial dentistry. The CDA was very sympathetic to this group and urged Ottawa to ensure adequate treatment. Members of the third class were not on relief, but could not afford dental care and went only when in great pain. The CDA complained that many practitioners were treating these people free of charge out of compassion, to the great detriment of their colleagues. The fourth class consisted of "wards" of the state who were generally receiving some form of dental treatment. Since the CDA thought that free treatment for everyone was impossible, the government should focus on children. It recommended that the Department of Pensions and National Health, in coordination with the provincial departments of health and education, give children yearly dental exams, along with education. If parents could not afford care, then Ottawa should provide treatment.[28] It also called for a federal dental division, under a dentist, at Pensions and National Health.

The Second World War

The war focused attention on dental health in Canada. As described above, 23 per cent of the men who enlisted were rejected because of dental defects. As a result, military officials changed the dental requirements and decided that it made more sense to fix recruits' teeth, which required a slew of dentists. By 1943, a quarter of the country's practitioners had signed up for the Royal Canadian Dental Corps, including more than 90 per cent of new graduates.[29] In the years just after the war, it became clear that the nation's dental health was not much better. The 1945 "Medical Survey of Nutrition in Newfoundland" (not then part of Canada), found that 40 per cent of people sixteen years of age or older had lost all or most of their teeth.[30] In Welland, on Ontario's Niagara Peninsula, the Red Cross discovered that only 20 per cent of children had ever seen a dentist and that the average child had five cavities.[31]

The realization of Canadians' poor dental health coincided with great enthusiasm for new social programs and government interventions. After relative wartime prosperity, people wanted to avoid the bleak conditions of the Depression. In 1943, Leonard Marsh's *Report on Social Security for Canada*, prepared for W.L. Mackenzie King's Liberal government, recommended cradle-to-grave social supports, including children's allowances, expanded old-age security, and medicare. It did not call for full dental coverage, indicating that the backlog of need was too great, but suggested providing dentistry for children through schools.[32] The Cooperative Commonwealth Federation (CCF), with its strong commitment to social welfare and a more equitable society, was gaining strength in opinion polls, threatening the ruling Liberal party. Bureaucrats and politicians alike embraced the reformist atmosphere. In the 1945 election campaign, all three parties included health insurance in their platforms.[33]

The CDA was convinced that publicly funded dentistry was on its way and in 1942 adopted a series of principles that would guide its provincial counterparts in their negotiations with the provinces for the next half-century. These principles spoke to dentists' pride in their profession, their confidence in their expertise, and their belief that professionalism required independence from the state. Dentistry, they said, should be carried out in the dentist's office, and any plan should involve the province's government and its dental board. Patients should have the right to choose their dentist, and vice versa. Preventive care was to have priority over restorative, and the profession would determine the need for its services.[34]

These demands resembled what Gregory Marchildon and Klaartje Schrijvers have described as "medical liberalism" among physicians in Canada and Belgium who resisted state encroachment after 1945.[35] In 1943, the CDA's submission to the federal Advisory Committee on Health Insurance (Heagerty Committee), which was exploring possible medical insurance, cautioned that the backlog of dental need and shortage of personnel made dental care for all Canadians impossible. It recommended focusing on children up to sixteen, and adding older people as resources became available.[36]

But many dentists opposed state-run care not just as impractical – they also feared losing their independence. As one of their leading figures, Donald Gullett, CDA secretary 1942–64, observed in 1943: "Any health insurance program must not encroach on private initiative … Canadians must be free to choose their own dentist [and] the dentist must be free to say what patients he will take." He added: "Mechanized service would be ruinous. You can't put the public on an assembly line."[37] Similarly, the dean of dentistry at the University of Toronto, Arnold D.A. Mason, warned that regimentation under any health plan would stifle the profession. Dentists, he said, were pleased to advise the government on providing services, but such projects should preserve competition. "If we ever become regimented we will kill off the type of man who may wish to enter dentistry"[38] And of course, the use of "man" was not accidental – that gender dominated the field.

Dentists' work with returning war veterans fuelled their opposition to government involvement. Aware of veterans' sacrifices, and eager to avoid the unrest that had followed the Great War, the government offered servicepeople comprehensive benefits, including dental. Civilian dentists, however, believed that they were not being paid enough for this work and resented what they saw as disrespect for their professional judgment. Military dentists examined members of the services before they were discharged and described the work they needed to seek from their family dentist. Civilian practitioners who disagreed with the diagnosis had to check with Ottawa or be denied payment. Numerous organizations, including the Toronto Academy of Dentistry, the Eastern Ontario Dental Association, the St Catharines' Dental Society, and the Manitoba Dental Association, also protested the fee schedule.[39]

Dentists closely followed Britain's evolving healthcare situation under the Labour government of Clement Attlee, elected a month after victory in Europe. Britain's new National Health Service (NHS), introduced in 1948, covered dentistry. The CDA sent its secretary, Don Gullett, over that year, and he mourned the loss of independence under the NHS. He thought the service focused too much on treatment, rather than prevention.[40] He reported that dentists were receiving very bad press, some members of the public were calling for lower incomes for them, and they were losing morale. After the NHS began, many people rushed to have their teeth fixed and obtain new dentures, and for a few years dentists were overwhelmed. Then, a revision to the act in 1951 forced patients to pay £1 towards treatment, and half the cost of dentures. Suddenly, patients dried up.[41] At the same time, the auditor general and comptroller accused dentists of "scamped work and even of fraud," leaving a black mark on the profession.[42] While Canadian dentists looked askance at the NHS experience, many British dentists remember it differently – a 2013 Witness seminar, which brought together people who had practised in this era, suggested that, despite policy changes, incomes remained high, and many patients received desperately needed care.[43] Overall, dentists in Canada felt that private practice guaranteed their status and independence, but also their income.

Many Canadian practitioners believed that people could afford their services if they budgeted better and prioritized their teeth. As an editorial in the *JCDA* stated: "Our people spend as much on candy and confections as on dentistry; half as much again on radios and musical instruments as on dentistry; half as much again on dog bills and veterinary fees; half as much again on jewelry and silverware; nearly twice as much on cosmetics as on dental service; over twice as much on liquor; over twice as much on sports and games; four times as much on tobacco; over four times as much on beer; five times as much on motion pictures and over fifteen times as much on automobiles, new and used, as on dental services."[44] As a result, practitioners showed little enthusiasm for any sort of dental insurance.

Despite the recommendations of the Heagerty Committee and the support of all three political parties, the plan for medical insurance floundered when the provincial governments refused to give up their powers of taxation to the federal government.[45] Meanwhile, Ottawa sought to educate people on how to take care of their teeth, as we saw in chapter 2. In 1945, National Health and Welfare set up a Dental Division, which concentrated on children. This of course made sense in a country experiencing an unprecedented postwar baby boom and focusing attention on children's health and welfare.

Postwar Possibilities

A major issue hindering public dental care in the 1950s and 1960s was the shortage of dentists. During the Depression, admissions to dental school plummeted. They began to recover after 1945, but the ratio of dentists to people was actually worsening. Immigration and the baby boom were expanding the population rapidly, and many practitioners were over fifty and retiring or nearing retirement.[46] By the mid-1950s, growing alarm finally led to action. The University of Toronto's Faculty of Dentistry received a major grant from the province to construct a new building and increase student numbers. The Faculty of Dentistry at Dalhousie opened a new home in 1958, doubling student places. Manitoba accepted its first class of dental students in 1958. The University of British Columbia's opened a dental school in 1965, and Faculties of Dentistry at Western Ontario and Saskatchewan accepted their first classes in 1966. In 1967, Laval in Quebec City announced plans for a dental school. By the mid-1970s, the ratio of dentists to people was much improved, and dentists, especially in urban areas, were beginning to complain that their practices were not busy enough.

Although government medical insurance failed to materialize in the 1940s, public support for the measure was strong, and the three parties continued to endorse it. In 1957, Parliament passed legislation giving the provinces matching funds to provide free hospital services. In 1961, John Diefenbaker's Conservative government appointed the Royal Commission on Health Services (Hall Commission) to investigate the possibility of funding physician care outside of the hospital setting. Three years later, the Hall Report recommended taxpayer-funded medical insurance for all Canadians. It advised implementing a dental program for children, using dentists and auxiliaries, as quickly as possible. It suggested starting with five- and six-year-olds and then expanding it each year, so as to cover all children 3–18 by 1980, by which time adults might be included as well. It also strongly urged dental services for expectant mothers.[47]

The CDA criticized the plan for offering too much treatment and not enough prevention. It opposed the dental plan for children, favouring health promotion and more dentists, and blasted the proposed use of auxiliaries to treat children. The CDA insisted: "It is naïve to think that good dental health for the children of Canada can be achieved by removing financial barriers to dental care. Factors other than economic impede the translation of dental need into demand. Long-established habits and attitudes must be overcome before the desired acceptance rate can be realized. This can only be accomplished by dynamic public health programs continually educating, inspecting and referring children for diagnostic, preventive and treatment services."[48] As well, the CDA stressed universal water fluoridation, dental education, and more dental research.[49]

By this time, the CDA much more strongly opposed the public provision of dental care. People's incomes had risen substantially since the 1930s, and dentists believed that most people could afford dental care if they were only willing to spend the money on it. In cities across Canada, fluoridation had been defeated in municipal referendums, sometimes repeatedly. Dentists interpreted the rejection as indifference to dental health.[50] In its own plan for young people, released in 1968, the CDA urged personal care for oral health and suggested that education and water fluoridation could vastly improve children's oral health. It wanted all young people to enrol in a voluntary pre-payment plan (in effect, insurance for future treatment) to cover care by a private dentist. To deal with the shortage of personnel in rural areas, it proposed incentives for opening practices outside cities and a guaranteed annual income from the state for practices treating a high proportion of children. It also urged training of many more dentists and dental hygienists.[51]

There was widespread agreement that large-scale denticare, even for children, would require a major increase in personnel, including auxiliary workers to make practice more efficient. Near the end of the Second World War, only about half of the practising dentists in Canada employed an assistant of any kind.[52] In the years after 1945, recognition grew that auxiliaries could increase efficiency. During the war, research showed massive gains in productivity by employing three chairs and a dental assistant. In the 1950s, US dental schools began pioneering the strategy of having two people working chairside, later known as "four handed dentistry."[53] Many practitioners began employing assistants to help them chairside, do clerical work, clean equipment, perform lab work, and so on. Often the dentist trained them, although the University of Toronto had begun a program for dental nurses in 1919.[54] Dental hygienists could further increase productivity by providing preventive procedures without the dentist in the room.

Many dentists were enthusiastic about the training of hygienists. Canada's first program started at the University of Toronto in 1951, but graduates were few, and, despite the interest in establishing programs at other universities, there was a shortage of space for training hygienists. Dalhousie and Alberta finally launched programs in 1961. The net result was that there were few highly qualified auxiliaries in Canada. Ontario in 1968 had only 306 dental hygienists, most of them in and around Toronto. In the mid-1970s, training moved to the province's community colleges, 11 of which had programs by 1977.[55] The cadre expanded: by 1978, Ontario had licensed 1,196 people. In 1971, the Université de Montréal offered a baccalaureate in dental hygiene, aiming to supply educators for Quebec's community colleges (CÉGEPS, originally *Collèges d'enseignement général et professionnel*, created in 1967). By 1975, there were dental-hygiene programs at seven CÉGEPS, including three in the Montreal area (one English and two French) and programs in Québec City, St-Hyacinthe, St-Jérôme, and Trois-Rivières.[56] But dental hygienists were allowed to practise only under a dentist's direct supervision, which limited their potential for providing oral health care in schools.[57] By the early 1970s, another concern was that their training took too long relative to the sort of patient care they were allowed to do.[58]

In 1966, Parliament passed the National Medicare Act, with funding starting two years later for provinces that set up medicare. By 1971, every province had done so, and many were considering dental care for children. Several sponsored commissions, studies, and special reports, and provincial dental associations put forward their own plans. The biggest stumbling block was the expense. Health economists and government bureaucrats soon noticed that medicare was substantially more costly than previously estimated. Politicians and health bureaucrats worried that dentistry would be very expensive. A number of studies proposed having auxiliaries take over some of dentists' tasks.[59]

National Health and Welfare's *Ad Hoc Committee on Dental Auxiliaries Report* (1970) received wide attention. It demonstrated that Canadians typically still had very poor oral health. Some of the best data came from new military recruits. Over 95 per cent of the men aged 17–23 had decayed teeth, and over 50 per cent had no fillings, indicating that they had visited the dentist only for extractions. More than 85 per cent had lost at least one tooth, and more than a third had or needed a full or partial denture. The report suggested that physicians were using auxiliaries far more effectively than dentists were. It listed four types of accepted dental auxiliaries in Canada: the dental hygienist (trained for two years at a recognized dental school and who performed education and prophylaxis); the dental assistant (often trained by the dentist to do office work and some chairside assistance); the dental receptionist / secretary; and the dental technician (who fabricated appliances, and many of whom trained as apprentices). In addition, there were dental mechanics (see chapter 5), New Zealand–type dental nurses (see next paragraph), and Canadian Forces therapists, who were trained by and could work only in the forces. These last, after three-and-a-half years doing duties similar to the dental hygienist, took 16 weeks' training on how to fill teeth prepared by the dental officer, take preliminary impressions, remove sutures, and irrigate post-operative wounds. They vastly increased dental productivity, although it was not clear if they would benefit civilian practices, which operated very differently.[60]

The *Ad Hoc Committee Report* of 1970 and numerous later studies looked at New Zealand's Dental Nurse Program, started in the 1920s.[61] When a reformist dentist, T.A. Hunter, took over the Dental Division of the country's Department of Health, he had just organized a dental corps for the armed forces. He had long been interested in dental care for children, and there had been much discussion about the need for a state dentistry program to improve the oral health of schoolchildren. Hunter decided to implement a full-time service in schools offering preventive and early corrective dental care. The island nation lacked the necessary dentists, but Hunter saw no need for them in a program that would use only part of their training and skills. In keeping with the maternalist ideologies of the era, he thought women "temperamentally and psychologically more suited than men to deal with and treat the ailments of young children." Hunter launched intensive training for young women to learn simple fillings, extraction, and preventive work, and the first nurses entered schools in 1923.[62] The program transformed the country's dental health. The number of extractions per year per 100 patients fell from 407 in 1922 to 19 in 1960. A 1968 study of young adults found that 55–75 per cent of their decayed teeth had been filled. (By comparison, only 20 per cent of the decayed teeth of Canada's military recruits of the same age were filled.[63]) The United Kingdom initiated a similar New Cross Auxiliary program in 1960. Graduates provided dental care to schoolchildren, though under closer supervision than New Zealand's dental nurses. Their two years of training taught them to fill, scale, clean, and polish teeth, extract deciduous (baby) teeth, apply fluoride, and teach oral health.[64] In both New Zealand and Britain, auxiliaries were widely accepted by children and their parents.

Canada's Ad Hoc Committee reported that once dentists in those countries saw the value of the auxiliaries, they usually received them well.[65] The committee also warned about a strong correlation between income and visits to a dentist and that removing financial barriers was not enough to encourage people to seek care. A study of a private US insurance program found that only 27 per cent of the families of skilled or unskilled workers used their pre-paid coverage over a period of five years, while 50–60 per cent of professional, sales, skilled, and executive employees did so.[66] The committee concluded that school dental services could improve the dental health of children quite dramatically and that school-based programs could reach the largest number of children. It advised that the use of auxiliaries would be necessary to provide a successful dental program for children.[67] This report set the stage for discussions in provinces about how to improve access to dental care, especially for children.

Children's Dental Programs

Access to dentistry for children in postwar Canada ended up varying widely: Newfoundland, Nova Scotia, Prince Edward Island, Quebec, Manitoba, and Saskatchewan all offered programs at various times. In other provinces, such as Ontario and British Columbia, municipalities did so. The program in North York (Toronto) was particularly extensive.[68] This section, rather than reviewing every province's story, explores the debates in those that acted – ironically, mostly those with a shortage of dentists. Dentists and policy-makers believed that such endeavours could attract new practitioners, particularly to underserved areas, as the extra income could provide the basis for a financially successful practice in these regions. In provinces with higher ratios of dentists to people, such as British Columbia, Alberta, and Ontario, most parents – except those on social assistance – paid for their children's dental care. The unwillingness of dentists to consider providing dental care outside of the private dental office meant that many children's dental programs exacerbated rural–urban inequalities, in that rural children were less likely to receive care than children living in urban areas with better access to dentists. This meant that rural taxpayers were subsidizing the dental treatment of the urban children who had access to care.

Newfoundland set up the first children's dental program for five-year-olds in communities that had a dentist in private practice – a significant caveat, because the new province had only one dentist for every 12,000 people, by far the worst ratio in Canada.[69] Its only practitioners were in the capital, St John's. In 1965, the program brought in six- and seven-year-olds, in 1971 all children zero to ten, and in 1978, eleven- and twelve-year-olds. In 1970, the program was extended to all children across the province.[70] By the early 1980s, it had a 50 per cent rate of use. The province's relative lack of dentists made it hard for patients to obtain care even if it was free.

Saskatchewan, also a majority rural province with few dentists, launched a much more innovative program. It founded a dental school in 1965, which had its first graduates in 1972.[71] Under the leadership of the Cooperative Commonwealth Federation (CCF, 1944–64) and the successor NDP (1971–82), the province had long been a pioneer in the provision of publicly funded health care. All this made the New Zealand model of children's dental care particularly attractive to Saskatchewan politicians. The government sent a delegation there in the early 1960s. One returning delegate, A.E. Chegwin, director of the Dental Health Division of the Department of Public Health, commended the program for its high-quality, comprehensive care.[72] The representative of the College of Dental Surgeons of Saskatchewan, orthodontist J.J. Schacter, condemned the program for its use of antiquated equipment and the poor quality of the training provided to the nurses, although he admitted the children's oral hygiene was excellent, the quality of their fillings was good, and the dental profession in New Zealand was very much in favour of the program. Schacter's biggest objection seemed to be to New Zealand's welfare state, which he said had "undermined the individual and has curbed his freedom," so that, for the sake of security, the New Zealander was willing to accept "mediocrity" – a clear indication of Schacter's political leanings.[73]

Many civil servants liked the idea: Deputy Minister of Health Dr Clarkson believed that dental nurses could ease the dental-health crisis among young people.[74] In 1966, Ross Thatcher's Liberal government announced a five-point program to solve the province's troubled oral health, including training dental therapists. That same year, the CCF platform called for denticare.[75] The College put forward an alternative plan based on prevention, not treatment: dental inspections at schools, with cards sent home indicating necessary treatment, and topical fluoride applications. The program would involve dental hygienists, dental-hygiene assistants, and clerks, all supervised by dentists, because, it maintained, people were not willing to receive treatment from people with "inferior (two-year training) if they have a choice." It argued that "dental nurses" stayed on the job for an average of only seven years, and that a study of dental nurses in Britain showed that they were significantly less productive than dentists. As a result, taxpayers should invest in training dentists.[76] But the province remained short of dentists into the 1980s. In 1971, a survey showed that at age seven, 76 per cent of children needed one or more teeth filled and 39 per cent required extractions. By age eleven, 40 per cent had gum disease, and about the same number had poor dental hygiene.[77]

In 1970, Saskatchewan started with a preliminary project for schoolchildren in the Oxbow region, supported by the federal government. It outfitted a 50-foot mobile home with three fully equipped dental operatories (working spaces), a waiting room, a staff room, and a bathroom, which moved among the region's schools. The staff included two British-trained dental therapists, a receptionist, a dental assistant, and a dentist.[78] Using the Oxbow data, in 1972 the Department of Health put forward a proposal for children 3–12. Dental auxiliaries would clean, scale, fill, and extract teeth, apply topical fluoride, and teach dental health. More complex cases would be referred to private practices, which would receive fees for services. To prepare for this, the Institute of Applied Arts and Sciences in Regina began training dental nurses in September 1972. In Saskatchewan, as elsewhere, some experts worried that dental nurses might be more expensive than predicted because women supposedly tended to drop out of the labour force. Public-health officials worried that their unique training program might lose alumnae to other provinces.[79] The department doubted that the program would reduce the incomes of dentists, who would still receive referrals for complex care. Also such services for children would eventually increase adult demand, as people saw their value.[80]

An advisory committee to the department led by K.J. Paynter, dean of the University of Saskatchewan's College of Dentistry, counselled that any children's program should emphasize prevention over treatment and urged the government to push for fluoridation and remove candy and pop machines from schools. It insisted on dentists providing all examinations and prescriptions for treatment in any free dental care, at least at the program's start. The advisory committee wanted dental nurses to be more fully supervised than the initial proposal suggested. It reported having received briefs suggesting treatment in private dental offices, but worried that this would add to costs. A committee member, dentist A.W. Giesthardt, submitted additional comments. He was highly critical of the plan and of the authors' failure to consult with the province's College of Dental Surgeons. He complained that parents opting out would pay twice: to the government, through taxes, and to their dentist. He wanted dental nurses closely supervised by a dentist, who should be available at all times. He also saw a role for dental hygienists: people trained in both treatment and prevention (i.e., dentists), he said, usually focus on the former; dental hygienists, trained in prevention, lack that tendency. He suspected that the program could undermine rural dentists financially and recommended surveying them in advance.[81] The next year, the *Ontario Dental Journal* published a scathing article condemning the competence of the dental nurses, the possible expense, and the paperwork involved.[82]

A 1973 report by Saskatchewan's College of Dental Surgeons opposed the proposal, called for more discussion, and added that the province would do better to legislate water fluoridation.[83] It maintained that any successful plan needed extensive consultation and collaboration with the profession. Dentists needed to be present during any treatment, such as preparing cavities, inserting fillings, or extracting teeth. A November 1972 survey of the College's members showed that 95.8 per cent favoured direct supervision by dentists. They argued that this would improve the work and would make better sense for the patient, as occasionally straightforward procedures prove more complex, perhaps beyond the capacity of the dental nurse.[84] The College's 1973 report was extremely patronizing towards the young women expected to become dental nurses, assuming that they would lack confidence and skill and be easily overwhelmed. The (male) dentist, it posited, could help relieve her fears and assist when she was lacking or in a medical emergency.[85]

The College's report asserted that most dental disease was preventable and that people should take care of their own oral health, and that the way to do this was to force parents to take their children to see a dentist.[86] It found New Zealand's dental-nurse plan out of step with current-day best practices and condemned the lack of opportunity for those nurses to upgrade their skills or training. It excoriated the schooling for Saskatchewan's dental nurses, judging the curriculum haphazard and the faculty as lacking teaching experience.[87] Incidentally, it insisted on only female dental nurses to prevent illegal practice. As we see in chapter 5, dentists believed that male auxiliaries, such as dental technicians, were far more likely to embark on illicit practice.[88] The report warned as well that the children's program might jeopardize rural dentists' practice and income.

Despite the reservations of the College and its advisory committee, the province's minister of health, Walter Smishek, believed in the proposal, and the government commenced the Saskatchewan Health Dental Plan in September 1974. It started with six-year-olds and gradually expanded to cover children five to sixteen by 1982–83. Most care was provided by dental nurses (later called "dental therapists"). In most locations, they travelled to clinics set up on school grounds.[89] The profession remained strongly opposed to the plan, although many members applied for its salaried positions.[90] The public, in contrast, supported it strongly. A survey in 1978 showed 89 per cent of parents satisfied, and only 7.8 per cent were unsatisfied.[91]

Opposition to the plan from the College continued, and in 1981 students at high schools in some urban areas with enough dentists were dropped from the program.[92] In 1987, the Conservative government abolished the Saskatchewan Health Dental Plan and created the Children's Dental Program, which covered dental care by private dentists, to be paid by the government on a fee-for-service basis.[93] Historian Garry Ewart sees this as an ideological decision – the savings were minimal and undid broad coverage.[94] Opposition to the closure was strong – thousands of residents marched on the legislature. The former NDP premier Allan Blakeney claimed that it was the province's largest protest in 25 years.[95] One excuse for ending the program: the province now had enough dentists. The closure was devastating for the 411 employees, including many specially trained dental therapists, now virtually unemployable.[96] (In 1978, legislation allowed dental nurses to work for dentists, partly because the government had trained too many of them. It had expected large numbers to marry and leave the workforce, but many remained on the job as more and more married women took work outside the home.)[97] Eventually, three former employees sued the government and the College. A lower court awarded them damages, later overturned.[98]

Quebec also introduced a children's dental program in 1974 – the government reimbursed dentists for care, which increased use of dental services. In 1975, only 25 per cent of young people visited a dentist; in 1981, 57.4 per cent.[99] Rates of use were much higher in urban areas, partly because dentists were scarce in rural areas. Most rural patients needed to wait more than four weeks for appointments. But, as Gilles Dussault explained, other factors inhibited dental care, including "negative attitudes towards dentists and dental procedures and other economic costs such as transportation or time out of work."[100] He criticized the children's program for downplaying prevention, noting that while more children's teeth were filled, the number of missing and filled children's teeth in Quebec were still way too high by national and international standards.[101] Problems with access also plagued Nova Scotia's program, launched in 1972. In the first four years, 85 dentists set up practice in the province, increasing the ratio of dentists to people and presumably access to private care.[102] Even so, by 1982, only 50 per cent of eligible children were receiving care.[103]

By contrast, Saskatchewan's plan enrolled 84 per cent of children in 1981–82, and others were receiving private care.[104] It was not expensive: the cost per child dropped dramatically from 1974 to 1986 through economies of scale and because the backlog of needed care had been addressed. The expense per young person enrolled or treated was similar to Nova Scotia and Newfoundland's, but quite a bit lower than Quebec's, even though only Saskatchewan's plan included administrative costs, suggesting that it was actually cheaper.[105] Malcolm Brown's costing of the Saskatchewan and Newfoundland systems concluded that the former enrolled more children and provided them with more and cheaper services.[106] Long travel times and the attention to preventive care added to its costs.[107] As James Leake pointed out in his study of options for Manitoba, the plans in Quebec and Nova Scotia were most successful in areas with many dentists and did not reach the children most in need of oral care.[108]

Ironically, just as Saskatchewan was reproducing New Zealand's model, Kiwis began to ask new questions about the effectiveness of the school dental service. As Susan Moffat has shown, a 1973 World Health Organization study showed that 36 per cent of its residents aged 35–44 had no teeth – the highest rate of all the countries surveyed. Nor had the school dental service eradicated socio-economic inequalities in oral health: rural and poorer residents were still worse off. Part of the problem was lack of access after students graduated. A complicating factor was the unfavourable image of the school dental clinics, often known as the Murder House. This may have discouraged adult New Zealanders from seeking oral health care as they aged.[109]

Despite Canada's notable interest in the New Zealand model, the dental nurse / dental therapist never became a large part of dental care in Canada. The Saskatchewan program lasted only 13 years. Manitoba used dental therapists in rural areas for just two years: the opposition of the Manitoba Dental Association persuaded the new Progressive Conservative government to replace the program with a fee-for-service plan, sending program staffers to provide community preventive services instead.[110] By the late 1980s, Manitoba provided dental care to rural children through a mix of private clinics and school-based programs. The school programs were cheaper to deliver and had higher rates of use.[111] Prince Edward Island employed dentists and dental hygienists trained in restorative work in a children's program. These "expanded duty" hygienists were able to help fill a cavity. As in Saskatchewan, children were treated in school-based clinics. Eligibility began to be cut in the early 1980s but was restored a few years later.[112] The program stopped making use of expanded-duty dental hygienists sometime after 1983, and by 1995 care was turned over to private dental offices.[113]

By the late 1970s, health economists in Canada and elsewhere were increasingly sceptical that public dental insurance could increase use. The less-than-stellar rates in Quebec and Nova Scotia were discouraging. It was clear that people with private insurance, increasingly common in the 1970s, did not always take full advantage of it, perhaps because of high co-payments or other factors, such as fear of dentists. A study of BC children with full coverage found that only 70 per cent visited the dentist in a given year.[114] Another concern of health economists was that people with the highest incomes tended to visit the dentist most frequently and spend a higher proportion of their income on dentistry, meaning that publicly funded services would benefit the rich more than the poor. While one might assume that these differences in use would ease if everyone was covered, they did not seem to be based entirely on ability to pay, since even studies of existing insurance plans showed that people with higher incomes tended to visit the dentist more often. As health economists R.G. Evans and M.F. Williamson explain in *Extending Canadian Health Insurance: Options for Pharmacare and Denticare* (1978), "A public dental insurance plan which did not significantly influence utilization rates would in fact serve to subsidize the relatively higher-income classes who now use the largest proportion of dental care." They suggested that unless incomes taxes were adjusted to tax the rich more, the net result might transfer wealth from poorer members of society to the wealthy.[115] They added that if denticare was intended to encourage people to use dental services, it was unlikely to work. A *BC Report on Children's Dental Health* suggested that insurance would raise use of dental services from 60 per cent to only 70 per cent, reaching only one-quarter of the children not already seeing a dentist.[116] A study comparing the children's programs in Saskatchewan, Quebec, Prince Edward Island, Nova Scotia, and Newfoundland noted that

Saskatchewan and Prince Edward Island increased use the most. The author concluded that fee-for-service programs benefitted primarily children whose parents would have taken them to the dentist regardless of cost. He further suggested that fee-for-service practitioners might be abusing the plan by offering more of the financially rewarding services, such as radiographs and oral hygiene instruction, compared to cheaper treatments, such as restorations.[117] The recessions of the early 1980s and early 1990s and the rise of neoliberalism resulted in cutbacks in children's dental programs across Canada. As we saw above, Saskatchewan cancelled its plan in 1987, although children were now insured for dentist visits, until that plan was cancelled in 1993. In 1982, Quebec stopped covering children 13–15 and preventive services for those under eleven. Nova Scotia ended coverage for children 10–11 in 1996, and additional cuts reduced coverage for fillings to low-income households.[118] No other provinces devised universal programs, although many continued dental public-health services such as education and fluoride rinses.

With the decline of government interest in funding dental care for young people, training of dental auxiliaries for children came to an end. By the 1980s, the shortage of dentists, which spurred thinking about alternative modes of service delivery, had eased. New dental schools and the rapid growth of dental hygiene as a profession meant more dentists and more efficient practices. The decline in children's cavities reduced the dental workload. Practitioners, especially in urban centres, needed more patients, making them even more hostile to programs that took business away from the private dental office. This was especially unfortunate for low-income children, who were the ones most likely to benefit from school programs.

Programs for People on Social Assistance

The other major category of patients covered by publicly funded dental insurance consisted of recipients of social assistance. Not surprisingly, Saskatchewan, Canada's postwar innovator in health policy, was the first province to cover such people.[119] Alberta soon followed, and by 1962 five provinces had such programs.[120] Quebec introduced its version in 1976, along with child denticare.[121] By the early 1980s, all of the provinces had coverage except Prince Edward Island, Nova Scotia, and Newfoundland, although Ontario's covered recipients only of Family Benefits (single parents, seniors, and persons with disabilities).[122] Social-service caseworkers in provinces without plans were able to authorize emergency dental treatment.[123]

One of the best-researched programs was the Ontario Dental Welfare Plan, which began in 1958 through an agreement between the province's Department of Public Welfare and the Royal College of Dental Surgeons of Ontario (RCDSO). Originally, it covered only children of beneficiaries under the provincial Mothers and Dependent Children Allowances Act. It was administered by the Canadian Dental Service Plans Incorporated, an insurance agency established by the profession, which agreed to provide basic services to designated beneficiaries. Initially, the province paid 70 cents per eligible beneficiary per month for basic services: examination, prophylaxis, restorations, and extractions. Patients had the free choice of dentists, who did not have to accept them. The plan was extended in 1963 to children aged 16–18, and in 1965 to parents. (Fathers became eligible when the Mother's Allowance Act gave way to the Family Benefits Act.) In 1966, the RCDSO began to reimburse dentists at 90 per cent of their fee schedule.

In the plan's first ten years, fewer than one-third of eligible residents actually used it.[124] In his 1969 study, James Leake showed that beneficiaries in regions with fewer dentists were less likely to enrol, suggesting problems with access to care. Also, the plan covered only basic care, and Leake argued that dentists disliked having to neglect proven procedures such as space maintainers, root-canal therapy, and dentures. Some also complained that welfare recipients were much more likely to break appointments. Leake suggested that a universal school-based program for children might better ensure that all Ontarians received similar care and oral health education.[125] In a 1970 study, economist Ron House observed: "There is little inducement for dentists to accept these beneficiaries and trouble has been experienced in attracting dentists to participate in the plan." Insured children up to sixteen received a card allowing them dental care paid by the province, but most dentists in Peterborough, for example, refused to accept these cards, denying the holders treatment.[126]

Dentists regularly complained about their low pay for these services. In 1968, for example, BC dentists (receiving 57 per cent of their fee schedule for such care) decided to offer only emergency treatment, leaving many people without care.[127] In 1969, the Association professionelle des chirurgiens dentistes du Québec, during its debate with the province over fees for services to people on social assistance wrote: "*Quant aux tariffs d'honoraires, c'est le statu quo de la loi de la jungle, celle du plus fort: on nous impose, d'une façon autocratique, des taux ridicules and inférieurs dans certains cas, au salaire horaire payé aux boueuers, aux plombiers, aux mécaniciens, aux électriciens.*"[128] Recipients of social assistance finally became eligible for dental care in 1976. By 1978, dentists were increasingly refusing to provide treatment and embarked on a campaign for higher fees.[129] Since the plan did not cover everything, some recipients, expecting free treatment, became angry at the dentist when told services were not insured. Practitioners claimed that they did not have time to explain treatments properly. Many thought that co-insurance, whereby patients paid part of the cost of the insurance, would encourage personal dental self-care, so deeply did they believe that oral health was up to the individual.[130]

The problem of access to care continues, as recent studies in Quebec have shown. People frequently do not make use of the available dental benefits. Recipients must wait a year after assistance begins for dental benefits to kick in, and many people use welfare sporadically, especially if they work seasonally. As well, benefits cover only a limited range of services, and, most notably, not root canals. Finally, some beneficiaries cannot find a dentist to treat them.

At the turn of the twenty-first century, a team of researchers in Montreal did one-on-one interviews with sixteen adults (aged 30–48) on welfare who had experienced a dental problem in the previous year, many of whom reported mental illness and addiction and / or domestic violence. Only one-eighth of the participants went to the dentist regularly. Of the eight participants in moderate pain, only two tried to visit a dentist. The first was refused service because her benefits were not yet available. For the second, the dentist recommended a root canal, which was not covered, so the person gave up. All of the six with severe pain went to a dentist. One had "crumbling teeth" but was turned down by several dentists as not yet eligible, and another was told to have a root canal, so she sought out a practitioner who would accept payment in instalments, but this effort took time. Eventually, she had a root canal, but there were complications, and the tooth had to be extracted. Participants had a variety of techniques for dealing with the pain: eating soft foods, using substances to numb the gums, alcohol, Tylenol, and removing the teeth themselves.

While patients seemed to be generally happy with their last treatment, they reported being suspicious of dentists and their motivations, believing that they recommended more profitable treatments. At least one was upset that her dentist reprimanded her for not taking care of her teeth. Several reported that they felt stigmatized by the dental office. The authors argue that, given the difficulty of paying for root canals, many patients and dentists opt for extraction. They conclude that interviewees "generally view dentists as rich people at the opposite end of the social scale who are not very sensitive to their problems; according to them ... motivated by financial interest more than by the health of their clients."[131]

Researchers have sometimes speculated that social class affects how people feel about their teeth and that this helps to explain why people on social assistance do not make full use of available services. For example, a 1970 study by economist Ron House for the Committee on the Healing Arts in Ontario concluded that poor people were unlikely to seek out dental care. "The key to improving dental health is individual motivation. Even if a mouth has been restored to health by treatment, neglect of proper oral hygiene and failure to seek further professional services soon will reduce the mouth to its former condition. When this occurs in a public dental health program the expenditure of community funds may be considered largely wasted."[132] But interviews in the early twenty-first century with recipients of social assistance in Montreal found that they highly valued having a nice smile (perhaps partly a reflection of the growth of cosmetic dentistry in the 1990s and beyond, which I trace in chapter 6). Interviewees saw a broad smile and white teeth as an indication of self-care and good health. One participant said, "Just watch television, they all have white teeth. Look at actors and actresses." Many considered white teeth essential to employment: "An interview for a job is all about appearance." They also thought it crucial for advancement in a career. Many were self-conscious about their own teeth, commenting on missing, crooked, or discoloured ones, which prevented them from socializing or seeking work. Many saw dentures as the only possible solution.[133]

Where differences among classes did emerge was in responsiveness to expert counsel. A Montreal study showed that parents who were recipients of social assistance managed their children's dental care confidently, based partially on their own experience. They often visually inspected their children's teeth for cavities and took them to the dentist when they were in pain. Baby teeth with cavities that did not hurt did not necessarily trigger a dentist visit – these would eventually fall out. Parents felt responsible for their children's oral health but managed it on their own terms.[134] Fear of dentists may be a bigger issue among recipients of social assistance than in the general population. Another study found it an obstacle to seeking dental care: "It scares me, so for me to go and see a dentist ... it really needs to hurt so much that I can't handle it, and there's nothing else [that can] be done!" Another reported, "When I have a toothache, my children tell me 'Mom, go to the dentist.' I'm not about to tell my children that I'm scared to go to the dentist. I tell them, 'Yeah, yeah, I'll go tomorrow.' I'll take some Tylenol ... I don't tell them I'm scared of the dentist ... They don't need to know that."[135]

Many of the same researchers showed why people on social assistance may have felt scared or patronized at the dental office. They interviewed thirty-three Montreal dentists. Many were irritated by how often people cancelled appointments and expressed frustration that they could not deliver the best care possible because public insurance restricted available treatments. And patients often had to turn down root canals that they could not afford, leading their caregivers to believe that they did not value their oral health. These practitioners hated extracting teeth that they could have saved. Many were angry that the government paid them so little for this work. They felt that they had to provide a different, lower level of care than they prided themselves on, and this conflicted with their sense of professionalism.[136]

These issues were not confined to Quebec. In the late 2000s, a study at the University of Toronto asked Canadian dentists about publicly funded dental care. Many resented the low fees and the onerous claims and adjudication. They wanted governments active in dental care, but in measures like water fluoridation, direct prevention, and oral health education. One of their major frustrations with public plans was the few services covered.[137] Given many dentists' lack of patience with patients on social assistance, and most of the recipients' anger about their treatment in dental offices, many of these patients prefer care in a publicly funded clinic or dental school, or even through hospital emergency departments.[138] But hospital care is expensive. It is also ineffective at solving the underlying dental problem as it generally consists of pain medication and antibiotics. Proper dental care would improve the quality of life of these patients.[139]

While every province has provided dentistry for people receiving social assistance, they have been reluctant to pay dentists at their full fee schedule, and there have been onerous claims processes that make dentists resentful towards governments and sometimes even patients. Patients themselves face obstacles to care, including dentists who refuse to take them, as well as personal issues, such as fear and shame about their teeth as well as caregiving obligations, addictions, and mental health problems that keep them from fulfilling appointments. As dental offices become more luxurious, that may also increase patients' unease. As a result, people on social assistance often do not take full advantage of available services. Different models of service provision, such as community clinics staffed by salaried dentists, might better serve this population.

Programs for the Disabled

In the early twentieth century, many institutions for the disabled provided some dental care, but staff members were not trained to offer basic oral hygiene, nor did they necessarily appreciate the value of keeping the teeth clean. Institutions often lacked dental staff, despite many patients' dire need. A survey published in 1971 found that only four of nineteen Canadian institutions for people with developmental disabilities had a full-time dentist, and many lacked a dental suite, so patients needed transport to a private office.[140] In British Columbia, the Woodlands Institution in New Westminster, now notorious for abuse of patients, had a dentist one day a week in 1916, and a full-time dentist in 1937. At first, the service did mostly extractions, but it expanded over time.[141] In other institutions as well, many children had their teeth extracted, instead of repaired.[142] This is very similar to what happened for Indigenous children in residential schools.[143]

It was not until the 1950s that dentistry for the disabled emerged as a field of practice.[144] At the University of Toronto, residents began treating children with special needs at the Hospital for Sick Children. The American Academy of Dentistry of the Handicapped was founded in the early 1950s and started a journal in 1974. That same year, Dr Norman Levine, a leader in dentistry for the disabled, and a professor at the University of Toronto's Faculty of Dentistry, opened the Mount Sinai Hospital Dental Program for Persons with Disabilities in Toronto.[145] Gradually, dental schools began adding material on the subject to their curriculum.[146] Even so, the Commission on Dental Accreditation of Canada still does not require that practitioners be qualified to provide care for adult patients with special needs.[147] In 2010, half of the country's dental schools still provided no instruction on how to treat patients with disabilities, who often need dental care more than other people.[148] Children with developmental disabilities often have more tooth decay because brushing their teeth is difficult.[149] Many people using wheelchairs use their mouths to hold things and do other tasks, compromising their oral health.[150] In her powerful report, *Help: Teeth Hurt!* (2013), disability activist Joan Rush described how many adults with development disabilities waited for up to two or three years for appropriate treatment. Since many of them cannot speak or write, they sometimes beat their heads or bite their arms because of dental pain: some have broken facial bones, while one man suffered a retinal detachment after smashing his head.[151]

The wave of de-institutionalization across Canada in the 1970s coincided with the emergence of children's dentistry programs in many provinces. Disabled youngsters in the community were often covered under such programs, and disabled adults under those for people on social assistance, including for people with disabilities. Even so, both children and adults, though ostensibly covered, found care difficult to obtain, as did people with disabilities who paid for dental care. Historically, many dental offices were inaccessible and did not accommodate wheelchairs.[152] Many dentists felt ill-at-ease treating patients with disabilities because they lacked the training.[153] Some felt frustrated by the extra time required.[154] After Woodlands closed in 1996, there was no attempt to provide a specialized clinic in New Westminster.[155] One study that asked parents in Saskatchewan about dental care for their disabled children found that while most were satisfied, some complained that their children were anxious in the dental office and that dentists "lost patience, became irritated and rushed the treatment."[156] Several studies of parents found that dental care was not a priority for them, as they had so many more pressing medical issues to attend to.[157]

Numerous studies have shown that people with disabilities find obtaining dental care a challenge, but the degree of difficulty has varied widely.[158] In 1971, an Ontario study reported 15.5 per cent of parents of children with Down syndrome and 25.9 per cent of parents of children with cerebral palsy found it difficult to arrange for dental care.[159] A more recent study discovered that 26.8 per cent of people with disabilities in Ontario experienced barriers to care, but these included personal barriers like fear of dental procedures and inability to express dental pain, as well as environmental factors such as cost, lack of transportation, physical accessibility, or dentists' refusal to treat them. Fewer than 10 per cent of people reported denial of treatment. Disabled people were actually more likely to have visited a dentist in the previous year than the general population. That said, the response rate was low, and perhaps included people who were more active about seeking treatment.[160] A survey of Ontario dentists in 2006 found that 80 per cent treated patients with special health-care needs, defined very broadly to include cancer, liver disease, and renal disease. Most had received relevant education, and 40 per cent had taken continuing education on the subject. Just under 40 per cent had patients with cerebral palsy, and almost 60 per cent had treated people with Down syndrome. However, only 52 per cent of dentists responded – probably those most interested.[161]

A 2004 study of parents of children with Down Syndrome found that these youngsters were more likely to see a dentist than their siblings who did not have Down Syndrome, but received less preventive care and had more teeth extracted.[162] According to a 2008 study of people with developmental disabilities, dentists were more likely to recommend extractions for disabled patients rather than major restorations. Caregivers complained that dentists were unwilling to provide dentures or orthodontic treatment.[163] Part of the problem is undoubtedly the very low fees paid to dentists for work they completed for people with disabilities. As dentist Clive Freeman explained in 2015, social assistance reimbursed practitioners at only 40–50 per cent of their normal fees. Since many had an overhead of 60–70 per cent, they were in fact subsidizing treatment.[164]

According to qualitative studies with disabled individuals, significant barriers remain, despite recent efforts to improve dentists' education and to make their offices more accessible. In-depth interviews with BC self-advocates and caregivers of adults with developmental disabilities indicated that many self-advocates felt excluded from treatment decisions and believed that they were given incomplete information, although many also reported positive and trusting relationships with their dental provider. Several parents and self-advocates criticized inadequate insurance coverage and costly treatment and resented long waits.[165] Wheelchair users in Montreal in a 2011–12 study noted that locating an accessible dental office was very difficult, and even some offices that claimed they were accessible were not, leading to disappointment when the prospective patients arrived for an appointment. Transportation services were not always punctual and reliable, frustrating patients and dentists alike. Some clinic washrooms were inaccessible. Counters at reception were often higher than patients' heads, and some credit-card terminals were unreachable. Transfer into clinic chairs was difficult for many patients, and staff lacked experience, making it nerve-wracking as well.[166] Clearly, some dentists need more training to treat people with disabilities and deserve better pay. Again, there may also be a role for salaried dentists in specially equipped clinics, and for mobile dentists or dental hygienists who visit patients.

Programs for the Elderly

While most provinces funding public dental treatment did so for children, Alberta targeted seniors. In 1973, the Alberta Health Care Insurance Plan began covering people over 65 and their spouses and dependants for care by both dentists and dental mechanics, who had been licensed to practice in that province since 1961.[167] At the beginning, dentists received roughly 90–95 per cent of their fee schedule, but by 1992, only about 50 per cent.[168] They could "extra bill" patients for their services, but dental mechanics could not. Utilization rates were quite low: 25–27 per cent in the first seven years (many seniors would have worn dentures, and denture-wearers rarely visit a dentist yearly). By 1992, usage had increased to 44 per cent, perhaps reflecting the growing number of seniors who had their own teeth. Many of those who needed dentures turned to a denturist, despite the fact that cost-saving was probably not an issue, or at least not in the plan's early years. Patients maybe preferred denturists, or were accustomed to visiting them.[169] By the mid-1990s, many younger seniors were using the plan, increasing costs.[170] In 1995, the Extended Health Benefit removed routine preventive care.[171] The Extended Health Benefit was cancelled at the turn of the century and replaced with Special Needs Assistance for Seniors, for those with low incomes.[172] By the mid-1990s, seniors' incomes had risen significantly, and policy-makers did not regard a universal program as a wise use of "scarce" health-care dollars.[173] Indeed, while other provinces covered low-income seniors, only Alberta ever had a universal program.

Conclusion

Dentists were crowing by the late 1970s that they were far luckier than doctors who had to practise under "the long arm of the state." CDA President Dr Roderick Moran reported: "I feel sorry for the poor beggars [doctors] myself." He elaborated: "A person prices himself according to what he feels he's worth, and if the public wants to pay, it's their choice." Moran regarded most of the provincial dental plans as a "disaster," arguing that if people had their dental care paid for, they would not take care of their own dental health. He suggested that some form of deductible (fee to be paid by the patient) might increase feelings of responsibility.[174] Art Stoyshin, the president of the Ontario Dental Association, told a legislative committee in 1978 that the province's public health insurance was being abused and that dentists were able to provide a superior service, since they were free of "government meddling."[175]

In the late 1970s, Calgary dentists touted that even though they made slightly less than doctors, they were still better off. Dr Michael Wasylchuk told the *Calgary Herald* that dentistry was still a "private enterprise" with limited "government interference." "Doctors," he said, "gave up their ability to be part of a free enterprise situation when they went into medicare. The government has taken away many of their rights." The executive director of the Alberta Medical Association agreed, "We look at them [dentists] with considerably envy … They are able to establish fees and collect them without the interference of a third party in their relationship with their patients."[176]

Indeed, dentists' relief at being spared such "state surveillance" may have spurred the huge increase in applications to dental school in the late 1960s and early 1970s.[177] Thanks in large part to the growth of private dental insurance, practitioners' incomes doubled from 1970 to 1977, while doctors' increased only 47 per cent, and the consumer price index 60 per cent. Dentists still did not make as much as physicians, but worked far fewer hours per week.[178] Many dentists long prided themselves on their independence, and many revel in their roles as small business owners as well as medical professionals.[179] This professional identity has made large numbers of them highly resistant to state dentistry and hindered the development of publicly funded dentistry in Canada.

But such resistance is not the only reason Canada lacks denticare. The rising cost of public health care, the shortage of dentists from the late 1940s to the 1970s, and experts' growing recognition that access would not improve oral health for all citizens also helped discourage its emergence. So did many dentists' unwillingness to use auxiliary personnel, such as dental therapists, and their opposition to practise outside the private dental office. The rise of private insurance, which I explore in the next chapter, allowed most people to gain access to dental care through their employee benefits. As a result, despite renewed attention to the inequalities of dental care today, the solution appears to be targeted programs to increase access for people with lower incomes and to improve conditions for groups that have previously had access to benefits, but for whom benefits alone were not enough to remove barriers to care such as those with disabilities. Although the NDP called for denticare in the 2019 and 2021 federal-election campaigns, universal coverage seems unlikely. Better programs for people on social assistance, and new programs for low-income individuals, are more realistic. Even so, it is hard not to long for something like the Saskatchewan Health Dental Plan, which introduced all young people to the benefits of regular dental care through the public schools.

4

Insuring Smiles

The Expansion of Dental Care and Its Limitations

Len James did not grow up visiting the dentist. But not long after he started working for General Motors in St Catharines, Ontario, in the late 1960s, his union negotiated dental benefits for its members. The number of dentists practising in the city skyrocketed. Now, workers like James and their family members could receive regular preventive care, not just rush to the dentist when they were suffering the agony of a toothache.[1] Private dental insurance became a common employee benefit in the 1970s, making care accessible to far more Canadians, while increasing disparities in access. After the explosion in private coverage in the late 1970s, the working poor were much less likely than members of the middle and upper classes to have any dental benefits, but not eligible for the coverage available to recipients of social assistance. At first, women's lesser participation in the workforce meant fewer had benefits than men, but today numbers are roughly proportional. Other ongoing inequities: many rural residents had to travel long distances for dental care, and many immigrants struggled to obtain care, especially in their early years in Canada. One lasting consequence of these gaps is emergency-room visits for dental care, which are ineffective and wasteful, as the care required is not available in hospitals.

Private Dental Insurance

Health insurance started in Canada with lodge and industrial-contract practice in the nineteenth century. During the Depression, a number of hospital-based insurance schemes developed, which eventually grew into the Blue Cross. During the late 1930s, doctors' organizations began to offer insurance for physician services. The goal was to avoid the menace of state control by developing an alternative to state medicine. By 1947, physician-controlled Associated Medical Services in Ontario had more than 40,000 subscribers. Manitoba and British Columbia had similar plans, and by the late 1950s nearly one-quarter of Canadians had non-profit medical care, which by then existed across the country. Private insurance plans grew too.[2] Ottawa's introduction of Hospital Insurance in 1957 and the Medical Care Act in 1966 replaced physician-controlled and private insurance, as the provinces provided medical care to their residents.

The demand for dental insurance never equalled that for hospital and medical insurance, giving the dentists more time to respond to growing state involvement in medical care. Dentists looked first at post-payment plans that would allow patients to pay retroactively for required treatment. This had the advantage of allowing patients to receive care when they needed it.[3] In December 1955, profession-controlled Saskatchewan Dental Services introduced the first such scheme, which allowed patients to pay for care on a monthly basis without interest.[4] Such programs emerged in Alberta and Ontario in the late 1950s. In 1959, Canadian Dental Service Plans Incorporated was established to provide administrative services for provincial plans for dental care. It was intended that these schemes would be operated by dental organizations, not by the state. In 1960, convinced that pre-payment (of a certain amount each year for dental care) was on its way, the Canadian Dental Association (CDA), wanting to keep it under the control of the profession, developed a statement of Principles for Prepayment Plans and provided a model for how they might work.[5] The first such plan was created for the Sheetmetal Workers International Association in 1966 and added to the union's existing medical coverage.[6] It was administered by the Credit Unions and Co-operatives Health Services Society of British Columbia.[7] The Alberta Dental Services Corporation developed a pre-paid plan in 1968, which provided dental care to organized groups of at least 25 people. The union or corporation had to agree to pay at least 50 per cent of the costs and normally covered 70 per cent. The plan paid for basic services, including exams, fillings, and extractions, as well as root canals, and partially covered crowns and bridges, but orthodontics was not included.[8] The following year, a new pre-paid plan covered all dental costs up to $100 per year.[9]

Despite these small efforts, the profession as a whole failed to act on pre-payment plans, and the private insurers moved into the gap. In the late 1960s, commercial insurance companies hit hard by provincial medicare began moving aggressively into the dental field.[10] By 1968, the CDA was reporting that the field of pre-payment "is dominated by the commercial carriers."[11] In 1969, the United Auto Workers (UAW) met with the CDA to report that it planned to prioritize dental insurance in negotiations with employers, and that it favoured profession-run plans.[12] But the profession failed to act, and by the early 1970s the CDA appeared to give up. Nor was it particularly enthusiastic about third-party insurers. Although the CDA and its provincial affiliates could see that change was coming, apparently dentists wanted to keep their practice exactly as it had always been, with patients paying directly for services. John E. Sparks, the UAW's senior medical-care consultant, would become a leading critic of the dental profession, including its failure to proactively embrace insurance programs that would have extended care to a much broader audience. In 1969, he scolded the CDA's annual meeting for dragging its feet and told its members that private insurers would take over the field. Part of the problem was professional pride and intransigence. For example, the Ontario Dental Association had a principle that the practitioner must not have to submit a treatment plan, X-rays, or diagnosis to a third party.[13]

Unlike other types of health insurance that cover unexpected illness, nearly everyone experiences dental disease, which is quite predictable. Much of the care is preventive. Although expenses can be high, they are rarely "catastrophic" (unlike in other types of medicine), and cost and timing are usually not a complete surprise.[14] This is why the profession preferred the term "pre-payment" to insurance.[15] Costs for dental insurance depend substantially on how many people enrol. Start-up costs can be high, as many people delay or avoid dentistal visits in the absence of benefits, creating pent-up demand. Costs can also increase when companies decide to downsize or employees are expecting to lose their jobs, as they may flock to receive care before benefits expire.[16]

Dental insurance became a major demand in union negotiations in Canada in the 1970s. One advantage, for both employers and workers, of adding dental benefits to compensation was that these benefits are not taxable.[17] In 1969, only 41,000 Canadians had dental insurance, but by 1976 almost three hundred thousand had coverage, with rates highest in British Columbia and Ontario.[18] BC unions had been the first in the country to push for these benefits, following the lead of their western US cousins.[19] By 1982, about two-thirds of collective agreements in Canada included dental benefits, and about 36 per cent of Canadians had coverage.[20] Rates of coverage continued to be highest in British Columbia and Ontario, although Alberta and Manitoba were also seeing growing numbers of insured workers.[21] Employers liked dental plans, because they were tax-free and resulted in regular payments to lots of individuals, rather than one-time payments to just a few.[22] Growth slowed in the 1980s, but by 1996–97 53 per cent of Canadians reported having private dental insurance.[23] By 2009, 68 per cent had access to it through employee benefits.[24]

Insured workers and their families now flocked to have their teeth fixed. Spending on dentistry mushroomed. In 1960, Canadians spent an average of $6.61 per year on the dentist. By 2008, this had grown to $361.62 in constant dollars. This increase reflects the fact that the number of people visiting a dentist on a yearly basis had gone up, but it also reflects the fact that the number of procedures and their cost had risen. The cost per user in 1960 dollars rose from $19.04 in 1970 to $77.30 in 2008.[25] Spending rose particularly in the 1970s and 1980s, suggesting the role of greater access to private dental plans.

The growth in insurance changed dentists' practice, often to their chagrin. Many resented the extra paperwork, though recognizing that the coverage expanded their patient numbers.[26] Dentists had been accustomed to setting their own fee schedules, believing that better dentists could charge more. But such an unregulated market made it difficult for insurance agencies to predict or control costs. Dentists were extremely reluctant to have those bodies control their work, but, according to Sparks, the UAW critic, the diverse array of procedures and uncertainty over optimal treatment made it imperative.[27] Disputes over X-rays were particularly heated.[28] Admittedly, Sparks was a severe critic of the profession. According to the *Globe and Mail*, "he characterized dentistry as a class-oriented cosmetic service geared to the promotion of teeth as a sex symbol. He went on to portray dentists as a closed corporation whose affluent and avaricious members pursue the dollar with single-minded zeal but are callously indifferent to the needs of a long-suffering public."[29] He further chided them for increasing their fees by 43 per cent from 1961 to 1968. This compared to 20 per cent for the consumer price index and 28 per cent for doctor's fees.[30]

Dental insurance did little to equalize access to dental care, as it covered usually the most privileged, well-protected workers. A 1980 survey found that 67.6 per cent of managers and professionals had insurance, compared to 59.5 per cent of office workers and 60.6 per cent of non-office employees.[31] In the *Canadian Health Measures Survey 2007–09*, 78.2 per cent of higher-income Canadians had private dental insurance, compared to 60.3 per cent of people with middle incomes, and 32.5 per cent of those with lower incomes. Immigrants were less likely to have coverage than people born in Canada. Non-Aboriginal people were more likely to be insured than Aboriginal people.[32] Initially, men and women differed widely in dental benefits. In 1991, only 46 per cent of women had dental and medical benefits, compared to 59 per cent of men. Even at the same occupational level, women had less coverage – for example, 9 per cent fewer female professionals or managers had insurance than their male counterparts.[33] But by 2007–09, the differences were small – 61.9 per cent of women versus 63.4 per cent of men.[34] Because health benefits are tax-free (except in Quebec beginning in 1993), dental insurance increases inequality: through their taxes, people who lack it are subsidizing those who have it.[35] As economist Robert Evans pointed out to the Royal Commission on the Future of Health Care in Canada (Romanow Commission, 2002), an untaxed employee benefit of $1,000 is worth $500 to a wealthy person (in the 50 per cent marginal tax bracket) but little to those who pay few or no taxes.[36] Moreover, the expansion in private dental insurance reduced pressure on governments to increase dental coverage.[37]

In the late 1970s and early 1980s, most plans covered preventive services such as diagnosis, teeth cleaning, and in-office fluoride treatments, as well as basic services such as fillings and extractions. They paid the dentist based on the fee schedules set up by the provincial dental association, or by the insurer. The insurance agency reimbursed patients for their costs or paid the dentist directly. Many insurers covered 100 per cent of costs. Plans varied on what constituted a basic and a major service. Some did not cover more extensive services like crowns and removal of wisdom teeth; only 40 per cent included dentures; less than a third, fixed bridges; and less than a quarter, orthodontics. Not all insured services were fully reimbursed. Orthodontic treatment often had a lifetime maximum, which was far less than the cost of braces.[38] By the 1980s, more expensive procedures, such as orthodontics and major restorations, were more likely to be included.[39]

As we saw above, dental spending more than doubled during the 1980s, vastly outpacing inflation. As a result, insured companies began investigating how to limit benefits. One option was reducing regular examinations from every six months to once a year. The six-month recall was not well supported by evidence. When the Canadian Auto Workers adopted the nine-month recall, costs dropped significantly. The insurance industry's *Benefits Canada* reported "no evidence of worsening in oral health of employees," although it did not explain how that was determined.[40] Other ways to save money included fewer X-rays and use of sealants, which could slash decay and hence costs.[41] Other possibilities included a yearly maximum or increasing co-payments for certain procedures.[42] Some companies dropped claims assignment (whereby dentists directly charged the insurer), which they found was increasing charges. One employer had half its workers paying their dental costs and then submitting the claim to the insurer, while the other half paid nothing up front – instead, the dentist was reimbursed by the insurance. When workers submitted claims they averaged $162; when dentists submitted claims, they averaged $270. The business communicated the difference to employees and dropped assigned claims. Costs decreased by 10 per cent, even though a negotiated increase in fees made procedures more costly.[43] Most insurers and employers believed that having workers submit claims directly constrained dentists' billing.[44] A number of insurance companies looked into investing in dental companies to provide pre-paid services; the dentist would agree to provide care for enrolled patients at a specified cost per person.[45] This coincided with the growth of large dental corporations such as Tridont, which leased spots in shopping malls to provide a more convenient, less intimidating experience for patients.[46] Tridont also posted its prices, the first dental office in Canada to do so.[47] By the mid-1980s, there was a growth in pre-paid plans. This allowed insurers to control costs, as insurees were visiting the dentist more frequently than anticipated and having a larger number of procedures.[48]

Dentists opposed capitation (i.e., being paid by the number of patients), which they felt would lower the standard of care. The Ontario Dental Association's newsletter observed: "It is our view that capitation does not mean cheaper dentistry; it means cheapened dentistry," so it urged its members to boycott that system.[49] A major US study showed that dentists working under that scheme did fewer root canals and bridges. Instead, their patients had to make do with partial dentures. The Ontario Dental Association worried that it would restrict a patient's choice of dentist.[50] Indeed, when the Alberta Union of Provincial Employees looked into starting to offer "denticare" by employing dentists directly, it suspected that many people would be reluctant to leave their family dentist.[51] Ultimately, capitation plans never became a large factor in the market.[52]

Efforts to control costs continued in the 1990s. A 1994 survey found that eight out of ten Canadian employers felt that they were paying too much for benefit plans.[53] They were hoping to add choice or flexibility, increase employees' premiums and deductibles, and/or allow them to opt out.[54] In the mid-1990s, flexible plans allowed people to choose benefits – often helpful for dual-income couples who had two sets of family benefits.[55] In 1994, the École des hautes études commerciales in Montreal found that the cost of its health benefits, including dental, had doubled in just four years and turned to a flexible plan instead.[56]

Costs of dental care were rising by the late 1990s partially because patients, as well as dentists, were demanding new treatments such as white fillings instead of amalgam, dental implants, and root canals.

Some insurance companies suspected that some dentists were over-using benefits.[57] They might replace working amalgam fillings with white fillings, provide unneeded routine fluoride treatments, change the service date on bills to avoid yearly maximums, modify the procedure code, or upgrade the service to something more complicated than what was provided. Insurers planned to do more audits of dentists' billing, send audit letters to patients to ensure that the services were provided, or rewrite the plan to accord with evidence-based practices.[58] In 1998, *Reader's Digest* published a highly critical investigation. Its journalist went to numerous dentists for assessment – some recommended almost no treatment, and others, over $10,000 of work.[59] At least one UBC dental researcher agreed, saying that practitioners were allowing insurance plans to dictate their work, leading to over-treatment.[60] He pointed out that a study of sealants showed many children receiving them on pre-molars unlikely to decay. Many people recognized that plans allowed for unnecessary treatment. For example, dentists often scheduled check-ups according to their patient's insurance plan, rather than need.[61] As well, cutbacks to provincial children's dental programs meant more family members required coverage. Insurers were also grasping that more people with benefits were visiting the dentist, revealing societal norms in flux.[62]

In the 1990s, insurers began fighting back against increases in dental fees.[63] When the Alberta Dental Association increased its fees about 2.5 per cent, the Alberta Employer Committee on Health Care complained that fees had increased by 42 per cent over the previous decade, much faster than in other provinces. As a result, some employers reduced or eliminated dental benefits. Others threatened managed care – i.e., they would contract with professionally run dental clinics.[64] Blue Cross developed a "Blue Preferred Plan" whereby practitioners accepted a 12 per cent reduction in fees so they could join a list for Blue Cross customers. Employers would urge workers to visit such dentists to save themselves money, and co-payments could possibly save employees money as well. But very few dentists joined the list. As a result of these pressures from insurance agencies, the Alberta Dental Association decided to stop publishing a fee guide, because, it alleged, insurance companies were inappropriately dictating the dentist–patient relationship. Without a fee guide, dentists could focus on patients' needs.[65]

In the 1990s, as governments across Canada scrambled to bring down deficits, some considered taxing health benefits. Federal Minister of Finance Allan MacEachen had considered this in 1981, but the backlash was intense, and he retreated.[66] Quebec began taxing dental benefits in 1993.[67] According to *Benefits Canada*, as many as a quarter of employees in large companies withdrew; others went from family to single coverage. Employers and insurers worried that younger workers would drop out, which would increase costs over the long term.[68] A subsequent analysis by an MIT economist suggested that nearly 20 per cent of firms in Canada stopped providing employee benefits.[69] In the mid-1990s, Ottawa explored taxing dental benefits, prompting a major CDA advertising campaign: "Enough is Enough: Taxing your health is *not* the way to solve Canada's economic problems."[70] In the end, the government decided against taxing the measure.[71]

Despite these changes, more Canadians were acquiring private dental insurance, but by 2010 100 per cent coverage was rare. Plans typically covered 80 per cent of basic services and 50 per cent of major services (such as crowns, bridgework, and dentures). The average yearly maximum was $1,500. According to one dentist, this top figure had remained unchanged since the late 1970s, resulting in an overall reduction in coverage.[72] Employers were reluctant to cut dental benefits altogether, because many workers use them, and they are popular.[73] During the 2000s, per-capita spending on dentistry increased significantly, but the amount covered by insurance dropped.[74]

Private coverage has allowed more Canadians access to oral health care. For example, according to the National Health Population Survey, in 1978–79, when dental insurance was first becoming common, 47 per cent of Canadians reported a dentist visit in the previous year; by 1996–97, the figure was 59 per cent.[75] Yet such insurance may have widened disparities. Access to it affects one's tendency to visit the dentist. In an early-1990s' telephone survey of Ontarians 50 and older, 46.7 per cent had insurance, with far less coverage among those 64 or older.[76] Many people lost coverage as they retired, or never had it – it became a widespread employee benefit only in the late 1970s. As for having seen a dentist in the previous year, 81.6 per cent of those 50–64 with coverage had done so, but only 69 per cent of those without. Visiting a dentist was also correlated with income – at $60,000 or more, the difference was minimal, but at lower levels it was significant – at less than $20,000 per year, 78.7 per cent of people with coverage had done so but only 62.8 of the uninsured.[77] A mid-1990s study in Quebec of the oral health of people aged 35–44 found similar disparities.[78] The National Health Population Survey 1996–97 found even more striking differences: 73 per cent of people with insurance had visited a dentist, compared to only 45 per cent of those without.[79] These disparities had an impact on health. In the *Canadian Health Measures Survey 2007–09*, uninsured respondents were much more likely to self-report fair or poor oral health.[80]

Private dental insurance increased access to care for many Canadians, but it left many working poor without. As more people acquired it, families like the Anables were left out. The Anables had seven children, two born with extra teeth that stuck out, leading them to be called "Fang" at school. But the parents could not afford orthodontic treatment. Mr Anable was a department-store janitor and did not have dental insurance. His spouse explained, "We just don't have the money ... You can get help on welfare or mother's allowance but a working man can't get any help."[81] She mourned that there used to be a Red Cross fund, but the money ran out a few years earlier. As Carlos Quiñonez and Rafael Figueiredo reveal in their aptly titled, "Sorry, Doctor, I Can't Afford the Root Canal, I Have a Job," public policies about dental care are highly moralized. Only people in dire need qualify for public insurance, while those who work are deemed able to care for themselves, but many cannot afford dental care.[82]

Dentists had mixed feelings about the new insurance regime. They objected to the control over their patient care and the additional paperwork. Yet by the 1980s, it had more than compensated for the loss of business caused by declining cavity rates.[83] As John Gillies, executive director of the Ontario Dental Association, observed, most practitioners now view it as a "mixed blessing." "We're prepared to live with the paper burden ... There are enough other benefits to it to make it worthwhile."[84] For patients with insurance, it significantly enlarged access to care, but facilitated over-treatment. It also increased inequalities: workers with higher incomes benefitted more from the tax break than those earning less, and working people without insurance were left behind altogether.

Rural Areas

Dental insurance was helpful only if the insured could find a dentist. In the quarter-century following the Second World War, in many parts of rural Canada, they were in short supply. As Sasha Mullally and David Wright show in *Foreign Practices*, physicians were often scarce as well, alleviated only by numbers of new immigrant doctors.[85] All of Canada's dental schools are located in cities. Students from rural areas make friends, establish relationships, and become part of the community in the cities where they train, and many want to stay there after they graduate. But this means that for rural residents it has often been difficult to obtain care. This chronic problem was of long standing but appears to have worsened in the postwar years, when there was a shortage of dentists across Canada and the country was urbanizing rapidly. In the 1950s and 1960s, most new graduates were reluctant to establish in rural areas, believing that they could make a better income and enjoy a more professional practice in a larger urban centre. Programs to lure dentists to rural areas had little success. The situation improved in the 1980s, however, when many large cities had a glut of dentists, so opening a practice elsewhere became more attractive. Even so, disparities continue today, with rural residents less likely to obtain routine care, even if they have dental insurance. Those who do go to the dentist often face barriers. Waiting times for appointments and distances to offices can be daunting. Parents need to take substantial time off work to convey their children to the dentist, and people with disabilities can often not locate an amenable dental office. As for Indigenous peoples in rural areas, the federal government refused to provide much dental care in the years before 1979, except on an extremely restricted basis, as Ian Mosby and I revealed in the *Canadian Historical Review*.[86] The federal Non-Insured Health Benefits Program (created 1979) has remained inefficient and inconsistent, so First Nations peoples are much more likely than their non-Indigenous counterparts to have their children suffer from early-childhood caries, experience oral pain, and lose teeth prematurely.[87]

The problem of care in rural areas was chronic. A Department of National Health and Welfare survey in 1948 found that 39 per cent of Canadians lived in cities with 10,000 or more inhabitants, and that these centres had 71 per cent of the country's dentists.[88] The ratio of dentists to people actually declined in the later 1940s and the 1950s, impeding recruitment of rural practitioners. There is no ideal ratio – it depends on how much treatment is required, how many people seek it out and for what services, and dentists' efficiency, but in the early 1960s the United States had one practitioner for every 1,900 people, and Canada one for every 3,000. The better-served Ontario and British Columbia had one for every 2,400, with far more in urban areas.[89] In British Columbia, in the 1950s, some rural areas had one for every 10,000 people.[90] In 1961, among communities with fewer than 10,000 residents, Manitoba had one practitioner for every 9,145 residents, Saskatchewan had one for every 8,411 residents, and Newfoundland one for every 30,859 residents. By comparison, in Ontario in communities with 10,000 or more people, there was one dentist for every 1,956 residents. Across the country, except in Newfoundland, which had long been short of dentists, every province had fewer than 2,700 people per dentist in places with 10,000 people or more.[91] In 1971, in Nova

Scotia, some counties, including Guysborough and Shelburne, had less than one dentist for every 10,000 people, while Halifax County, which included the eponymous city, had one for every 2,887. Nearly half of the province's dentists practised in that county.[92]

This general rural shortfall meant some appallingly bad oral health. This reflected not just lack of dental care. Poverty was also a factor. When dental hygienist Mary Pelletier visited rural northern New Brunswick in the mid-1970s, she reported, "The dental decay was unbelievable. I mean, we were right down to the little nubbies. The baby bottle syndrome (early childhood caries) was awful but it wasn't milk in the bottle. The nurses would tell us, 'Oh, they put some Coke in there and crunch up some cheesies.' I was like, 'Oh my God, the poor little children.' It was desperate." Many of these homes did not have flush toilets, and definitely could not afford oral care. "A toothbrush for the whole family was more normal than everyone having their own. This is the honest to goodness truth. We would go and give them each a toothbrush. We did a little presentation depending on where I was and what part of the province it was. When I look back on it now, I can't believe I worked in those conditions. When the child would say, 'Yes, we have one toothbrush for all of us.'"[93]

In the absence of dentists, some rural communities in Canada tolerated illegal practices. In Nanton, Alberta, an older but unqualified missionary dentist set up shop. When the province tried to stop him in 1959, the Nanton Economic Council was outraged: "If no other dentist was available, and Mr. Lewis suited the people who went to him voluntarily, why should anyone complain?"[94] Its support probably reflects the virtual impossibility of recruiting anyone else. Such a gap could also lead to serious complications. In the early 1960s, Bobcaygeon, a town in Ontario's Kawartha region now made famous by the Tragically Hip, had no practitioner. The nearest one was in Fenelon Falls – quite a trek. Ian Montagnes reported for the *Globe and Mail*: "In a town without a dentist of its own, regular examinations are onerous and toothache is endemic. As a result, one 17-year-old girl and several other young people just out of their teens have full sets of dentures."[95] Students missed a lot of school while travelling for dental appointments, and doctors were forced to do tooth extractions. One young girl failed to go to the dentist, and eventually an abscess spread to her brain and left her developmentally delayed.[96]

Part of the underlying problem was lack of dental schools or lack of space in them. As we saw in chapter 1, Canada's first dental schools were in Toronto (1875), Montreal (1892), Halifax (1908), and Edmonton (1918). Montreal's later evolved into two – one at McGill and one at

Université de Montréal. The University of Toronto's was much larger than the others, preparing nearly half of all Canada's dental students. Dalhousie was small – often graduating fewer than 10 students per year.[97] Not surprisingly, in 1961, Ontario had one of the country's best ratios of dentists to people, as did Alberta. There were fewer in the Maritime provinces and Saskatchewan, and shockingly few in Newfoundland.[98]

As chapter 3 explained, things began to change with the opening of new schools and the enlarging of others: the University of Manitoba opened a school in 1958, while a new building allowed Toronto's to expand.[99] The Universities of Saskatchewan and Western Ontario opened their doors in 1965, and the University of British Columbia graduated its first class in 1968.[100] From 1962 to 1984, the number of dentists in Canada more than doubled, from 5,999 to 12,624.[101] This would eventually help to alleviate the shortage, at least in major urban centres, but many people were gaining dental insurance, and more were going to the dentist regularly.

The problem was not just space. In the 1950s and early 1960s, dentists were desperately needed, but few people were applying to dental schools.[102] A special report for the Royal Commission on Health Services (Hall Commission) revealed that in 1962 the vast majority (75 per cent) of all qualified students were accepted. A number of schools, including Montréal, Manitoba, and Alberta, accepted virtually all qualified applicants, while McGill and Toronto were more competitive.[103] It is unclear why few students chose the field, although dentists complained about their salaries. In 1957, the *Saskatoon Star Phoenix* reported on average incomes of five groups of professionals: consulting engineers and architects received $14,581 per year, doctors and surgeons, $13,978, and dentists came in lowest, at $10,234, with teachers making just as much.[104] In 1961, the CDA created a National Recruitment Committee. A survey found that dentists believed that too few students were choosing the field because of incomes too low relative to workload and hours, "lack of public appreciation of dental services," the cost of the education and establishing a practice, and fear of "socialized dentistry."[105]

In any case, incomes rose rapidly in the 1950s and 1960s. From 1953 to 1963, the net incomes of private practitioners doubled.[106] In 1959, tax statistics indicated that dentists were the country's fourth-highest-paid profession, after physicians and surgeons, engineers and architects, and lawyers and notaries. That said, the gap between lawyers (at $14,123 per year) and dentists ($11,605) was significant.[107] Since 1949, dentists had seen the largest increase in average income of all the professions.[108] Even so, many felt poorly paid: in a 1961 survey, 82.1 per cent said that they would encourage a young person to think about dentistry as a career.

But among those who advised against, 41.5 per cent cited "adequate income."[109] But by the early 1970s, dental schools were flooded.[110] This might have had something to do with rising incomes, but it was also tied to the fact that the large, postwar baby-boom generation was attending universities, and seeking professional careers in greater numbers than previous generations. It may also be that dentistry became more appealing in an era of 'socialized" medicine, as we saw in chapter 3. In 1979, the dean of dentistry at the University of Toronto indicated that the faculty accepted only 125 of the 800 or 900 "serious and qualified" applicants.[111] Indeed, the increase in applications to dental schools may have begun in the mid-1960s, when the oldest baby boomers entered university. A study of applications to Canadian medical and dental schools in 1965–66 revealed that competition was tougher for dental than for medical schools, although 90 per cent of people who applied to both fields and were accepted by both chose medicine, suggesting medicine still seemed more prestigious and desirable.[112] According to a mid-1960s' editorial in the *Journal of the Canadian Dental Association*, although applications had increased, the quality of the applicants had not.[113]

Why were dentists reluctant to establish practice in rural communities? Before 1945, one issue was access to appropriate equipment and amenities. In rural Saskatchewan in the 1940s, lack of running water and sewage would make work a "drudgery."[114] Also, many dentists believed that rural people were not as likely to engage in preventive care or to go to the dentist, making their job more difficult.[115] Some worried about possible lack of patients and anticipated more income in larger centres.[116] Indeed, the CDA's 1963 Survey of Dental Practice found that places with 100,000–250,000 people offered the most income. Dentists in towns with fewer than 1,000 residents made about half as much as colleagues in mid-sized cities.[117] New dentists were worried about being far from continuing educational opportunities and from senior colleagues whom they could consult on tricky cases.[118] Some students dreaded the visibility and lack of privacy of providing health care in a smaller community. An editorial in the *Journal of the Canadian Dental Association* in 1974 suggested that dentists did not want to practise in rural areas because they could not make as much money, partially because jealousy from neighbours worked to keep incomes down. Another factor was that in smaller communities everyone knew each other and it was impossible to escape from patients, who would be omnipresent. The editorial writer complained: "Just find ways for the rural dentist to enjoy some private social life sometimes without even one patient reminding him in front of everyone present that cold water still hurts his tooth."[119] But as the number of dentists increased, students became more willing to consider smaller centres. In 1984, the CDA reported that recent applicants to dental school expressed interest in communities smaller than their hometowns, although it is unclear if they fulfilled these intentions after graduation.[120]

In the years after the Second World War, provinces tried to entice dentists to rural areas with bursaries and other subsidies. In the early 1950s, British Columbia offered grants-in-aid to attract practitioners to small rural communities that lacked a dentist and travel grants to help them develop a practice.[121] Such bursaries expanded after 1945, and by 1972, every province except British Columbia, Alberta, and New Brunswick had bursary programs to encourage dental students to open a practice in underserved areas.[122] In the 1960s, Manitoba offered a student bursary and a civil-service job for any dentist willing to travel. It supported dentists who wanted to practise on a per-diem basis using portable equipment and would provide supplies and assistants. But, according to C.H. McCormick, director of the province's Dental Health Care Services, these incentives failed.[123] Prince Edward Island offered interest-free loans to encourage students to take dentistry.[124] New Brunswick started bursaries in 1970, offering $6,000 in return for agreeing to work four years in an underserved area. In its first nine years, it had only thirty takers.[125] In 1959, Saskatchewan started a rural bursary to persuade its dental students enrolled out of province to return after graduation.[126] Even as it opened its own dental school, it expanded the program to any Canadian student who agreed to practise in the province. It also paid graduates $5,000 (later increased to $20,000) and provided offices and transportation for the dentist and "*his*" family, an indication that they expected the dentist to be male.[127] In the early 1970s, practice grants were also available in Manitoba, Ontario, New Brunswick, Prince Edward Island, and Newfoundland.[128] In 1974, Nova Scotia began offering $8,000 to dentists who would locate or relocate to designated areas, and an income subsidy of up to $5,000 per year.[129] Incentive grants encouraged communities to help set up dental facilities.[130]

In the 1960s and 1970s, Ontario gave bursaries to students who promised to practise in a rural area, but not all the bursaries were taken. Perhaps they were not generous enough – in 1963, they were only $1,000 for every year the student promised to serve in a rural community.[131] By the 1970s, too many dentists were taking the money and not fulfilling their obligation to practise in a rural community. Instead, the province planned to establish practice grants and a guaranteed annual income.[132] The bursary program worked, however, for Dr Jerry Asling of Hanover, Ontario. Although he grew up closer to Toronto, he received a provincial bursary for his studies in exchange for setting up a rural practice. He was drawn to the number of patients needing care in Hanover, close to Lake Huron. When he set up in 1966, matters were so urgent that he did full-mouth extractions (i.e., all of the patient's teeth) at the nearby hospitals on his "days off."[133]

In the early 1960s, the Ontario Dental Association carried out a recruitment campaign that targeted rural students. It took fifty students with high grades from eastern Ontario to tour Toronto's dental faculty and stay overnight in dentists' homes. It also invited guidance teachers to visit the faculty.[134] In the early 1960s, Saskatchewan tried to recruit dentists in Britain, with little success.[135] Newfoundland tried to entice British dentists in the mid-1970s, and seven travelled over to "take a look," although it is unclear whether any migrated.[136] This is strikingly different from the highly successful recruitment of British physicians to Canada – many were eager to escape the National Health Service (NHS).[137] By contrast, for their dental cousins, the NHS proved a bonanza right at home.[138] It is unclear why governments did not try harder to recruit overseas talent, but perhaps the shortage seemed less pressing than the doctor shortage, especially since dentists and many politicians tended to see dental care as a private matter.

Another option for neglected communities was mobile dentistry. In Saskatchewan in the early 1960s, two Regional Boards of Health employed full-time dentists, providing them with mobile clinics to take to smaller communities.[139] Beginning in 1969, Dalhousie University in Halifax provided a summer dental service, employing students to treat children in Tatamagouche, on the Northumberland Strait. It used a vacant classroom as a clinic. In New Germany (close to Bridgewater) in the summer of 1972, a mobile trailer was constructed to provide care; the clinic then moved to Terence Bay (not far from Halifax).[140] That autumn, the Nova Scotia Dental Association transferred the trailer to Guysborough County, where many people had never had access to extensive dental services.[141] In the mid-1970s, the BC Department of Health equipped mobile dental units for Prince Rupert, the Queen Charlotte Islands (now Haida Gwaii), and the district of Mackenzie.[142] Beginning in the 1970s, the University of Alberta sent summer students in a mobile dental clinic to the province's north to work under the supervision of a faculty member; it hoped that some might set up practice there.[143] Ontario used dental rail cars extensively, but these were cramped and hard to staff.[144] They were still operating in the 1970s, but one MPP complained that some communities were visited only once every seven years.[145] Across Canada, many dentists were happy to travel and work for a short period when they were young, or willing to go away for a few weeks or months at a time, but ultimately most wanted to remain in one place.

In the early 1970s, the focus intensified on the scarcity of rural health-care providers.[146] This was partly an issue of justice: according to the federal government, medical care was supposed to be equally provided to all Canadians, free of charge, but if rural people could not obtain it, then they were essentially subsidizing the health care of urban residents through their tax dollars. While dental care was not free for most people, the same injustices occurred when it was publicly funded. In Quebec, which covered social-service recipients and children, rates of use were much higher in urban areas. As dental researcher Gilles Dussault noted in 1984: "Unless efforts are made to improve access to dental care in peripheral areas and to encourage potential users to use them, only the well-to-do areas will benefit from services paid by tax from all regions."[147]

As greater numbers of dentists graduated in the 1970s, the problem began to diminish. Realizing that large urban markets were almost saturated, recent graduates were more willing to consider smaller cities.[148] Some established satellite practices in places too small to support a full-timer but needing a dentist one or two days a week.[149] Children's dental programs based on private practice, like those in Quebec, Nova Scotia, and Newfoundland, made setting up in a rural area less risky, with these young patients guaranteeing some income. Similarly, in rural Saskatchewan, one of the objections to the Saskatchewan Health Dental Plan (see chapter 3) was that it might remove rural children from the private roster, thereby making a rural practice even less feasible. Private dental insurance also helped to make practice outside cities more profitable, as more and more Canadians visited the dentist regularly, even though rural residents were somewhat less likely to have insurance.[150] It may have been easier for some families to obtain dental care in the 1970s, as having two cars became increasingly common, facilitating access.[151]

In Saskatchewan, cancellation of the provincial dental plan in 1987 exacerbated rural issues, as the children in many communities had been served by dental therapists, lessening the burden on parents to travel to cities for their youngsters' dental care. Some dentists who had worked with the program occasionally decided to stop going to these communities, where they had treated adults as well as young people.[152] Dental therapists asked to be allowed to establish offices to ease the shortage, but this was not granted.[153] In the summer of 1980, the government agreed to provide dentists in rural areas (anywhere outside Saskatoon and Regina) with grants of $800 per month to employ a fourth-year dental student, expecting the dentists to match the grant. Quite a few of these "externs" eventually chose to practise in rural areas, but this did not have a noticeable effect on where Saskatchewan dental graduates as a whole decided to practice; it seems the students who chose rural externships were people who were likely to open up a rural practice in any case, so the program was cancelled in 1988.[154]

By the 1980s, rural–urban disparities had eased. In Prince George, a northern BC city with about 70,000 residents, dentist Larry Anderson reported that, until the late 1980s, "we were overworked," but by the mid-1990s "nobody's overworked."[155] The Nova Scotia Dental Association's executive director indicated that by 1986 fewer communities were requesting dentists, and new graduates were finding it harder to identify locations to set up a viable practice.[156] Most urban areas had a surplus, and dentists were more willing to consider more rural settings. The New Brunswick Dental Society's executive director, Dr John Thompson, said that farm communities still found dentists difficult to recruit, but no resident was more than 40 miles (64 kilometres) from a dentist. By contrast, in Newfoundland, many outport communities were accessible only by boat and plane. Dr Toby Goshue, executive director of the Newfoundland Dental Association, reported: "In some areas ... it is still safe to say that proper dental care doesn't exist."[157] In the Canadian north, Indigenous peoples in rural areas were particularly likely to be underserved. In 1980, when urban dentists began complaining about the oversaturated market, the Northwest Territories was still in desperate need.[158] But, by the 1980s, the lively discussion about the rural shortage of health-care providers had quieted. As Canada became more urban and more diverse, discussions of health inequality shifted away from urban–rural divides to other types of inequality, including immigrants' health. Even so, in 2009, the dentist-to-people ratio remained 3.5 times lower in rural Canada than in urban areas.

Dentists continued to express unease about rural practice. On that front, a 2015 Université de Montréal study of the attitudes of graduating students towards rural practice showed that they worried about privacy and jealousy there – one reported: " [You tell your rural patients that dental treatment] will cost $5000 and it's expensive for them. Then in [*sic*] the weekend, when you want to do the cruise on your private boat, they will judge you for having a beautiful luxurious life."[159] But others felt that rural practice might be slower-paced and offer greater sense of community.[160] Some were drawn to making a difference. As part of his degree program at the University of Alberta, Berland Hammond needed to work at a satellite clinic in a northern community. He became convinced that he could really contribute in the north: "I see more decayed and rotten teeth in a day than most dentists in the city see in a month."[161]

The shortage continues to affect care in some parts of the country. According to the 2001 Canadian Community Health Survey, urban residents with dental insurance were more likely to make use of it than rural residents.[162] A 2016 study that mapped dentists in Quebec found that 90.3 per cent of the dental workforce was located in urban-census subdivisions. Only 0.3 per cent of dentists and specialists worked in non-metropolitan-influenced zones. In northern Quebec, Minganie–Basee Côté Nord, and the Gaspé Peninsula, residents travel long distances for oral health care.[163] A recent study of rural residents in western Quebec reported long waits for dental care – up to 1½ or 2 years for an appointment. Others indicated that the local dentist would not accept patients on welfare or with disabilities, forcing them to travel further for care. Transportation was an additional issue for many patients. One interviewee, who had travelled to a community close to Montreal for treatment for her child, reported: "Worth every penny it cost for transport and the night we had to spend there. Rural areas are not equipped for children or anyone that has a disability or is scared of a dentist chair." Patients also felt that they had no recourse for poor service – because everybody knows everybody, word would get around.[164] Another Quebec study found rural residents almost as likely to see a dentist as urban residents, but less likely to have routine check-ups and much more likely to report physical pain and / or psychological discomfort as a result of their oral health.[165] A 2006 Saskatchewan study discovered that rural women were just as likely as their urban counterparts to have visited a dentist in the previous two years, but rural men were far less likely (62.6 per cent v. 71.4 per cent, respectively) than their city cousins to have seen a dentist.[166] In Manitoba in the years around 2000, extractions under general anaesthesia were much more common in rural communities, especially in the north. In Burntwood Regional Health Authority in the far north, nearly one-tenth of children under five had surgery for early-childhood caries, compared to about one in 100 in Winnipeg.[167] In short, while media attention to urban–rural disparities in health care has diminished, and the growing number of dental professionals has reduced the gap in care, inequalities continue.

Immigrants

Until quite recently, dental researchers paid little attention to immigrant groups. An early investigation, in 1987, showed that at age five, newly arrived children in Toronto had more than twice as many cavities as non-immigrant children. A later study found cavities particularly common in certain ethnic groups.[168] In 1995, a report in North York (Toronto) showed that immigration was a risk factor for youngsters likely to suffer from early-childhood caries. Both children born outside Canada and those with immigrant parents were at higher risk.[169] Other studies have confirmed this.[170] Many immigrant families do not have a family dentist because they lack insurance.[171] Indeed, for immigrants of all ages, lack of insurance seems one of the most notable barriers to oral health care. Research on immigrant mothers in Montreal showed that few recent newcomers without insurance visited a dentist for preventive services (44 per cent), compared to those with public insurance (68 per cent) or private (71 per cent). Among immigrants who have been in Canada for more than ten years, 62 per cent were likely to visit a dentist if they had no coverage, 50 per cent if they had public coverage, and 82 per cent if they had private coverage. Immigrants, especially from visible minorities, are less likely to be union members than other workers, which affects their access to dental insurance.[172]

A major trend in the recent literature is declining oral health in the first few years after immigration, but improvement as people's incomes and language skills increase, the stresses of their resettling begin to ease, and they come to understand more clearly how health care is delivered in Canada. The immigration system, which recruits healthy and well-educated people, means that newcomers typically arrive with better health than the average Canadian.[173] But their health soon declines, because of the stresses of immigration.[174] One study of people who immigrated more than ten years earlier found them more likely to visit a dentist than native-born Canadians, suggesting that any negative affect is temporary.[175] More recent research showed a notable decline in immigrants' self-reported oral health in the first four years after arrival, even though at the time of migration they reported better oral health than the average Canadian. The authors blame immigration stresses and possibly new norms about oral health, meaning that immigrants are less likely to rate their oral health as excellent after being in Canada for some time.[176]

There are also significant differences among immigrants. Europeans are more likely to visit a dentist regularly than newcomers from elsewhere. More affluent immigrants were less likely to have unmet dental needs, as were those with greater proficiency in English or French.[177] A 2015 study of African immigrant children (aged twenty-one to seventy-two months) in Edmonton pointed out that many new arrivals from that continent are refugees (45 per cent) and struggle more with English, have less education than most new arrivals, and are more likely to lack the supports provided by chain migration. Many of the children studied had never been to a dentist (52 per cent), and the majority (63.7 per cent) had untreated caries, which is a much higher average than Canadian children.[178] A 2014 investigation of Bhutanese refugees and immigrants in Halifax reported that the majority of both the immigrants (53 per cent) and the refugees (85 per cent) had untreated tooth decay, and most of the immigrants (89 per cent) and refugees (98 per cent) had moderate to severe gingivitis. Their rates are much higher than those for the general population and speak to the fact that they also reported visiting dentists much less frequently than average.[179] A study of older Chinese immigrants in seven cities in Canada found that more than half did not obtain any dental services in the previous year. They were less likely to use dental services if they were older, lived in Quebec, had poorer health, had been in Canada for a shorter period, or had poor social supports.[180]

Many immigrants now seek dental care on trips to their homeland. Among elderly Chinese immigrants in Vancouver and Melbourne, many do not like visiting dentists in Canada or Australia because of the language barrier and cost.[181] Chinese immigrants in Montreal also frequently sought dental treatment in China, frustrated by the high cost and short hours of dental practice in Canada, and a feeling that the care in China was superior.[182] A letter to the editor of *Canadian Immigrant* noted: "Dentists in China, India, Malaysia, Singapore, Africa, the Arab world and beyond do the treatment right away for an amazingly cheaper price," and it suggested that Canadian dentists should provide "an easy, fast and affordable" treatment.[183] A study of Brazilian immigrants found that they faced barriers to access, including low incomes, language barriers, and their lack of knowledge about oral health care in Canada.[184] They too tended to seek care in their homeland. A 2015 study showed that 12.9 per cent of immigrants received dental care in their native country in the four years after arriving in Canada, especially if they lacked dental insurance.[185] Although the oral health of immigrants only recently became a focus of research, disparities have long existed, especially among the uninsured. Targeted programs could likely improve the oral health of immigrant populations.

Emergency-Room Visits

Because of the gaps in coverage, many people visit the emergency room for dental care. At a recent event sponsored by the Coalition for Dentalcare, which lobbies for universal dental insurance, emergency-room physician Dr Hasan Sheikh explained that he sees patients almost every shift who would be better served by a dentist. He described a typical interaction: "I see someone pacing around their emergency department room, they are usually holding their cheek, they are in a ton of pain and before I can even get to my introduction, who I am and why I'm there, they are already saying 'Doc, I need something for this excruciating pain.' The frustrating thing is that I know they need to see a dentist; they know they need to see a dentist and they knew that before they came to the emergency department but they come because they have nowhere else to go." Sheikh reported that some of these patients have no insurance, while others do but have been unable to find a dentist.[186] A telephone survey by Carlos Quiñonez in 2008 found that more than 5 per cent of Canadians have visited an emergency department for a dental problem not related to trauma.[187] Another study found that between 2003 and 2005, Ontario had 141,365 emergency-room visits for dental problems. These visits are expensive and usually only relieve pain, and do little to resolve the underlying problem.[188] From 2006 to 2014, numbers of such fruitless expeditions trended upwards, especially for residents of neighbourhoods with lower incomes, immigrants, and rural people.[189] A 2017 study estimated that such visits cost the Canadian health-care system $1.8 billion per year, money that could help plug gaps in care in a more effective way.[190]

Conclusion

Employer-provided dental benefits were a boon for dentists and patients alike. While dentists chafed at the restrictions and the additional paperwork, insurance benefits brought many new patients to their offices. Far more Canadians could now afford consistent preventive care, and the oral health of most people has dramatically improved. Despite cuts to many plans in the 1980s and 1990s, dental insurance ushered in a new era of regular dental visits for those lucky enough to have it. But not everyone obtained it, and even some who did still faced obstacles. The working poor have been particularly disadvantaged. Dental benefits are most common for executives and well-paid unionized workers. Fewer retail and service workers have insurance, and the skyrocketing costs of dental care add further obstacles. Also, as the oral health of the population as a whole improves, missing, crooked, or chipped teeth become more noticeable, and more of a liability for those left out. While the ratio of dentists to people has increased, some rural residents still travel long distances for treatment, especially for specialist care. Finally, new immigrants can encounter obstacles: many are not familiar with the delivery of health care in Canada, some do not speak the language, many cannot afford the expense, and some come from countries where regular dental treatment is not as common as it is here. While this situation seems to ease for people over time, targeted programs could still help immigrants maintain their oral health immediately after immigrating to Canada.

5

Aging Smiles

Dentures, Implants, and Keeping Teeth for a Lifetime

In 1994, the Vancouver journalist Nadine Jones explained what tooth loss meant to her: "As a teen, I suffered the tortures of the damned as my soft enameled teeth fell apart one by one. We couldn't afford $2 for fillings, so my mother paid $1 to have each tooth pulled. We called that 'dental care' when we seniors were kids during the Depression." She elaborated: "At the best of times, false teeth are a grind. Most of us with manufactured smiles have been embarrassed in an exclusive restaurant when a tomato seed became inextricably lodged under our bottom plate. Or we were forced to use Crazy Glue as a temporary measure to stick a tooth back in a denture before an important date. (Or adhesive tape that got soggier by the minute before Crazy Glue was invented.)" She added: "Even intrepid souls hate seeing their mates' teeth smiling at them from a glass of water beside the bed!"[1] In 1950, two Freudian dentists emphasized the psychological costs of dentures: "To some people dentures represent advancing age, an unwelcome change in appearance … a loss of strength, virility and sexual power. Many jokes refer to this linkage. Dentures may activate latent conflicts and emphasize feelings of inferiority. Here again, loss of teeth is clearly linked to loss of sexuality."[2] While they may have overdone the Freudianism, many of their patients probably did see dentures as a loss and an unwelcome sign of aging, although others, after years of pain, embraced their dentures. And as uncomfortable and distressing as these devices could be, they were arguably not as bad as not having them or missing one. As one patient put it, "These dentures are like a fickle lover. Sometimes they hurt you; other times they make you happy. They can make you glad, mad or sad. They often embarrass you in company. You can't live without them, with them you are miserable."[3] Or as one elderly woman mourned in the 1990s, "I never go anywhere without my teeth, I just feel terrible without teeth."[4]

For much of the twentieth century, Canadians expected to lose their teeth as they aged. As a joke, many grandfathers frightened young children by taking out their teeth. After a lifetime of pain and agonizing treatments, extraction came as a relief for some. But even then, adjusting to life without teeth was not easy. People's dentures clicked as they talked: a dead giveaway that they had lost their teeth. They made the wearer's cheeks sag and made them look older. Sometimes they fell out in social situations. Many people worried about bad breath, and poor cleaning made "denture breath" common. Some older people ate mostly soft foods – tea and toast – because their dentures hurt when they had to chew vigorously. Reduced chewing ability hampered mastication, and this caused digestive problems as well as risk of choking. Chewing releases the flavours in food and upper dentures covered many taste buds, so denture wearers experienced less pleasure from their food. Some wearers, especially those with hearing loss, found it difficult to enunciate clearly. Mouth sores, burning mouth, and headaches were common when dentures did not fit properly. Some wearers gave up dentures because of irritation or gagging.[5]

Today, a growing number of Canadians, especially those from the upper and middle classes, expect to have smiles that last a lifetime. Some of their teeth may be implants or fixed bridges – but they will work and look much better than the dentures worn by their parents and grandparents, thanks to improved oral hygiene and much more extensive dental treatment. These gleaming smiles are part of the pressure placed on the elderly, particularly women, to look young in a youth-centric society.[6] Certainly, keeping one's teeth involves a lot of self-care and time and expense at the dentist. But better teeth are not just cosmetic: they allow people to eat more nutritiously, enjoy food more, and have a better quality of life. This chapter explores the fight to recognize denturism as a health profession, the growing interest in geriatric dentistry in the later twentieth century, and the development of dental implants, which have enabled many older people to keep their teeth (or at least a much better facsimile of their own teeth).

Maintaining teeth was part of a much larger revolution in oral self-care, including regular brushing and flossing, professional cleanings, and restorative care, such as fillings, root canals, bridges, and, most recently, implants. As we saw in chapter 1, it was only in the 1920s and 1930s that most Canadians began brushing teeth daily. The belief that infected teeth caused rheumatism and heart disease led to many extractions. The interwar mania for pulling teeth meant that many people born around 1900 reached their older years (sometimes even middle age) without teeth. By contrast, many children born after 1945 drank fluoridated water, used fluoride toothpastes, and benefitted from a wide range of oral health programs. Then, in the 1970s, as many baby boomers started working, private dental insurance became widespread, making accessible the preventive care that can make teeth last for life. These dramatic improvements affected most of the era's children and younger adults.

Indeed, dentists showed little interest in aging patients until the 1970s. An article in the *Journal of the Canadian Dental Association* (*JCDA*) in 1949 indicated that most were "inclined to neglect denture work," finding it unpleasant and "unclear."[7] Articles on dentures stressed that both parties needed patience to fit dentures well and help wearers feel comfortable.[8] In a 1965 editorial, the *JCDA* announced, "Because they [senior citizens] consider tooth loss inevitable and because they do not sufficiently value their natural teeth, the majority of these people do not visit a dentist regularly, do not avoid cariogenic foods and do not brush their teeth as often as they should." The journal suggested that the profession focus on developing "proper dental health habits in childhood."[9] In a late-1970s survey, more than half of BC dentists found making complete dentures unrewarding.[10] Indeed, undergraduate textbooks on dentures, both complete and partial, stressed how difficult recipients could be and urged patience and empathy.[11] Another sign of the emphasis placed on children in this period is the number of specialists. In 1975, Ontario had 332 specialists: 137 orthodontists (treating mostly children), 32 paedodontists (who specialized in children), 52 periodontists (gum disease), and 20 endodontists (root canals). In short, far more specialists dedicated themselves to child patients than treated older patients.[12]

Before dental benefits became widespread, many people saw dentures as inevitable and believed that people with tooth trouble were better off replacing them with false teeth. Wealthier people were more likely to esteem preventive and reparative dentistry. We lack Canadian evidence, but in 1959 the National Opinion Research Center in Chicago asked respondents whether a 31-year-old married man with two children should spend $600 to have his teeth restored to good condition or spend $300 to have his remaining teeth extracted and dentures made. Of participants earning $7,000 a year or more, 63 per cent favoured restoration, but among those earning less than $2,000, only 34 per cent agreed. Age affected responses: clearly, attitudes towards dental care were changing. Only 32 per cent of people over 65 chose fixing the teeth, but 61 per cent of those 20–24.[13] Moreover, even if everyone had opted for expensive treatment, there were not enough dentists.

As I outlined in chapter 3, after 1945 dentists were keen to figure out how to make their services more efficient. Prior to the war, many had employed assistants, usually women, whom they trained to answer the phone, make appointments, and maintain records – some assisted chairside. Indeed, as Tracey L. Adams shows, dentists were counselled to hire only women, as early in the century many of the men in illegal dental practice had initially been trained as assistants.[14] Some practitioners hired dental nurses, graduates of a one-year program at the University of Toronto. But the organized profession saw the wave of the future in dental hygienists, who had training in prevention and could help with scaling and prophylaxis. Crowded dental faculties trained very few hygienists until the 1970s. Even so, dentists insisted that the necessary personnel could come from training more dentists and female assistants or hygienists – although these latter were not the field's only auxiliaries. Many, if not most, dentists had technicians make prosthetic devices, although technicians and dentists rarely shared space. There was undoubtedly a gendered component to this. Dentists were, at least in theory, eager to hire young women, despite reservations by some about non-dentists doing work inside the patient's mouth. In contrast, few asked technicians – mostly men – to work on their premises. Solo practice was still the norm, and most dentists could not afford a full-time technician, provide enough work, or supply adequate space. Many found it more pleasant to have female staff. In a patriarchal era, when men were used to commanding women, female workers seemed easier to control and manage. But there was another group eager to provide dental care and believed its members qualified – denturists.

Denturists

The people who came to be known as denturists usually started as dental technicians. Until the 1960s, when a number of community colleges launched programs, dental technicians trained primarily as apprentices, although some joined the Canadian Dental Corps during the Second World War.[15] Beginning in the 1930s, a number of people, whom I refer to as denturists, argued that they did all the work preparing dentures for clients while the dentist did almost nothing. They believed themselves more skilled at the task than dentists, because they specialized in the process and could provide cheaper dentures. They sought the right to work directly for the public. Dentists disagreed, claiming that fitting dentures was very complicated and involved tricky issues of oral health outside technicians' expertise.

This debate played out in numerous provinces, often becoming a major political issue. The denturists, though few in number, often had strong support from members of the public who had positive experiences with them, thought dentists were over-charging, and resented dentists' seeming arrogance and sense of privilege. Like chiropractors, who fought similar struggles and also received strong popular support, denturists proved skilled organizers and lobbyists and won considerable backing.[16] Not surprisingly, they achieved independent practice first in the west, where populism was strongest.

The Denturist Controversy

Sharon Lorah, 31, had been suffering from tooth pain for several years when her husband finally persuaded her in 1974 to have all her teeth pulled. She had been put under anaesthetic at Northwestern General Hospital in Toronto, when Dr Gerald Baker, an oral surgeon, asked her who had made the dentures beside her bed. She told him it was a denturist. He slammed down the lid of the dentures and reportedly gave her a twenty-minute lecture on why she should not go to a "dental mechanic."[17] He refused to fit her with the false teeth made by a denturist, and the operation was cancelled.[18] Lorah had recently moved to Toronto from Vancouver, where denturism was perfectly legal. She was outraged, and an embarrassed Ontario Dental Association agreed to cover the cost of her care, although it insisted that Baker was right in refusing to treat her. It is not known why Lorah decided to go to a denturist rather than a dentist, but it is likely that cost was a factor: she paid $125 for her dentures at a Scarborough dental clinic. By contrast, dentists usually charged $225–$350.[19]

In 1960, there were about 1,720 people working in dental laboratories in Canada. Many were in small labs; some were self-employed. In large facilities, relatively few technical workers were registered dental technicians. Many were immigrants trained in Europe. Quite a few were female – 17.5 per cent across Canada.[20] The technicians were poorly organized: one province reported 60 registered technicians, but the provincial association claimed more than 200. Another province's association had 400, with an additional 200 "working illegally and more or less openly."[21] Moreover, illegal practice carried little stigma: in one provincial technician's association, the vice-president had been convicted twice of illegal practice, and other members five or six times.[22] In the 1950s, some technicians began arguing for the right to deal directly with the public and called themselves "dental mechanics."

Eventually, "denturist" described the people who dealt with the public, and "technician," those who made dentures using a dentist's prescription. Some observers suspected that it was primarily armed-forces trainees who practised illegally, although a history of denturism in Alberta that relied heavily on oral testimony suggests a variety of backgrounds.[23]

The first campaigns to recognize denturism started in the west. In Alberta in 1931, two popular denturists, who had been convicted of practising dentistry illegally, launched a petition to have dental mechanics legally recognized. They received almost 6,000 signatures.[24] In 1933, the province amended its Public Health Regulations to allow dentists to associate with a dental mechanic by registering with the board and outlining the mechanic's tasks. Many such associated mechanics worked directly for the public and had little contact with the dentist. In 1958, a group of mechanics asked an MLA to introduce a private members' bill to provide them with their own act. The bill died, but a committee was established to study the situation; composed of members of the dental faculty, mechanics, government officials, and dentists, it could reach no agreement. In 1961, the Certified Dental Mechanics Act and the Dental Technicians Act recognized respectively dental mechanics, who made dentures directly for the public, and dental technicians, who made dentures and other prosthetic devices for the profession.[25] The president of the Alberta Dental Association was dismayed that the vast majority of governing Social Credit MLAS supported the denturists and complained: "Our presentations before the private bills committee could not stem this emotional anti-professionalism which exists in the rank and file of our government. Excellence means nothing – cost everything."[26] The legislation required that patients provide a dentist-issued certificate of oral health to the mechanic, a provision dropped in 1972.[27]

In British Columbia in 1954, dental labs carried out an advertising campaign in the newspapers saying that they provided a service equal to that of a dentist and they did so at lower cost. They complained that they did all the work of producing the dentures, yet dentists received the profit. The College of Dental Surgeons retorted that allowing untrained individuals "to interfere with the tissues of the human body" was dangerous.[28] In 1955, a provincial bill would have allowed dental technicians to deal directly with the public. The Dental Laboratory Association and the Royal College of Dentists of British Columbia opposed the move. The bill was referred to a special committee and never returned. Three years later, another bill would have allowed the same thing, but because of opposition from organized dentistry and some dental labs, this provision failed to pass. Instead, a Board of

Examiners was established to determine dental technicians' duties and scope of practice. Subsequent regulations permitted those who had worked illegally for at least seven years to deal directly with the public. The rules aimed to limit their numbers in the hope that the practice would die out, but rewarded those who had been practising illegally. In 1961, the BC Supreme Court struck them down.[29] In 1962, a new act recognized two fields of practice: dental technicians worked with the dentist's prescription, and dental mechanics could make dentures directly for patients who provided a certificate of oral health signed by a dentist or physician.[30]

Quebec allowed denturism in 1973. In the province with the highest rate of edentulism (toothlessness), illegal practice was widespread. Although dentists opposed the legislation, it passed with little opposition as part of a wider revisioning of the health professions.[31] As in other provinces, the patient needed to provide a certificate of oral health. Denturologists took a three-year CÉGEP program and needed to pass an exam for a permit to practise.[32] By 1996, denturists made more than 65 per cent of all dentures and partial plates in the province.[33]

In Ontario, the issue became particularly contentious, especially as the ruling Progressive Conservatives were divided and inconsistent on the issue. Also, in the 1950s and 1960s, the province's Royal College of Dental Surgeons had cracked down quite successfully on illegal practice by dental technicians, much more so than elsewhere in Canada, which made the denturists' demands for recognition all the more sudden and surprising. As well, the Ontario Dental Association (ODA), much larger and better organized than many of its provincial counterparts, ran a long campaign against the denturists.

Denturists first tried to organize in 1966 under long-time union organizer Lowie (Red) Rosen. ODA President Dr Ashley Lindsay denounced the denturists, claiming that many had not finished even the eighth grade. He warned that an ill-fitting denture could cause "excruciating pain in the jaw joints. It can destroy the bony ridges it sits on," and the irritation could even lead to cancer. The Governing Board of the Dental Technicians also opposed the denturists: "The people agitating for denturism are a disgruntled few who can't earn a living as technicians so want to be allowed to deal directly with the public."[34]

In 1970, the Denturist Society of Ontario was established, and several practitioners opened clinics. In response, the Ontario Provincial Police and the Royal College of Dental Surgeons raided several denturists' offices, seizing business records and equipment.[35] The denturists agreed to give $100 a month to their society to plead their case, and they hired a lobbyist, Gordon Smith, who had worked with denturist groups in Manitoba and Saskatchewan. Copying their Manitoba counterparts, the denturists ran full-page newspaper ads seeking public support. The province's leading dailies, the *Toronto Star* and Toronto's *Globe and Mail*, supported the denturists. The *Globe and Mail* pointed out that other provinces had already licensed them and argued that such specialists were probably better at making dentures than dentists, who did a much broader range of tasks.[36] The denturists received support from even major players in the dental field. Conservative MPP and Woodstock orthodontist Harry Parrot chastised denturists' illegal practice but said that it was time for dentists to accept them – too many patients were going untreated.[37] In 1972, government legislation would have allowed "dental technologists" to deal with the public directly.[38] The dental profession lobbied heavily against the bill, and the government withdrew it and appointed a committee to advise it on standards for denturists. The committee (which had no denturists) recommended a compulsory three-year course.[39] Worried that the training would cost too much, the government abandoned the plan and introduced a new bill that prohibited denturists from dealing directly with the public. Existing dental technicians or denturists could qualify to become dental therapists through exams, although even then they would still need a dentist's supervision. In the meantime, the Royal College of Dental Surgeons agreed to establish dental clinics that would provide low-cost dentures to the public. In response, the denturists bused more than 800 patients to Queen's Park to protest the legislation, which a standing committee debated for more than ten hours.[40]

Ben Sweet, the president of the Denturist Society of Ontario, announced that he would rather go to jail than work under a dentist's supervision. The denturists formed a citizens' committee to help them defeat the legislation.[41] In early 1973, the government set up the examinations and refresher courses to allow denturists to qualify as dental therapists. It held back on prosecution in order to give people time to qualify. Denturists felt that the deck was stacked against them, as the exam would be administered by dentists. In March, they indicated that they would refuse to take the exam. The opposition regularly attacked the government for its mismanagement of the situation and expressed concern that few dentists were providing dentures for $180, which the bill had promised.

In early June 1973, Health Minister Richard Potter hinted that he might back down on the legislation, as it was looking unenforceable.[42] But by month's end, he announced that he would proclaim it, knowing that 33 men had passed the qualifying exam and that the Royal College had agreed to cooperate in enforcement. None of the men who passed the exam belonged to the denturist society.[43] By the autumn of 1973, it was clear that the denturists were continuing to practise in defiance of the law.[44]

In early 1974, the province began its crackdown, staging raids on six denture clinics in Metro Toronto. One of the denturists was eventually charged and convicted of practising dentistry illegally. In addition to making dentures, he had fitted orthodontic bands on the teeth of an 11-year-old boy, suggesting that dentists' suspicions about denturists might be valid.[45] But then a major cabinet shuffle replaced Health Minister Richard Potter with Frank Miller. Miller quickly hinted that he would revisit the legislation, and in May 1974 he introduced a bill to allow denture therapists to put in full plates, but not partials.[46] Neither side was entirely pleased, but the legislation ended the conflict that had dumped masses of mail on the desks of provincial legislators and often preoccupied their chamber. Illegal practice continued. In 1980, Ben Sweet, the long-time president of the Denturist Society, served fourteen days in jail for making a partial denture. Only in 1993 could denturists legally make partial dentures.[47]

By the late 1980s, denturists were licensed to practice in every province except Prince Edward Island.[48] By 1999, Canada had roughly 2,000 registered denturists, nearly half of them in Quebec, where rates of edentulism remained the highest.[49] Ontario and Alberta accounted for the bulk of the rest.[50] The struggle to gain access to treatment by denturists was led by working-class people who found dentistry overly expensive and preferred the services of a denturist, as well as by the denturists themselves, who believed they provided a cheaper, better service. Today, many denturists argue that they offer a more specialized, more personalized experience than a dentist.[51] The dentists, by contrast, believed that their training in biological dentistry uniquely qualified them to work directly in the mouth. In essence, it was a challenge over expertise. Ever since the rise of professionalism in the nineteenth century, the professions have fiercely guarded their territories, and have often done so using the language of public safety. As Tracey L. Adams demonstrates in her recent *Regulating Professions*, legislators have been most sympathetic to the professions (law, medicine) whose members sat in legislatures and who had friendships and shared status with elected officials. But other groups able to mobilize support from patients, such as chiropractors and drugless healers, also obtained professional status.[52] Until very recently the male-dominated denturists have been far more successful in gaining the right to practice independently than the female-dominated dental hygienists, which parallels the experience of male-dominated chiropractors and female-dominated physiotherapists.[53]

Geriatric Dentistry

In the 1970s, a growing "grey power" movement brought attention to the needs of older people in Canada.[54] During that decade, the field of gerontology grew rapidly.[55] This had an impact in dentistry as well, and dental researchers began studies of the oral health needs of the elderly that painted a dismal picture.[56] A 1971 look at three seniors' homes in London, Ontario, reported: "In the past, most elderly people were resigned to any dental discomfort, and many still are. They have been the profession's forgotten people." Sixty-one per cent of the residents in their sixties had no natural teeth, as did 80 per cent in their seventies and 77 per cent in their eighties. Many were managing poorly fitting dentures with do-it-yourself denture re-liners or "wads of facial tissues."[57] Research in 1975 at Thamesview Lodge, a home for the aged in Chatham, Ontario, with many people who came from farming backgrounds, found 76.4 per cent edentulous. Appallingly, 46 per cent of those who needed a lower denture did not have one, while 37 per cent of those requiring an upper lacked it. Moreover, only 29 per cent of the upper dentures and 7 per cent of the lowers were ranked as in good condition. Of the people who still had some teeth, many required fillings and others needed extractions.[58]

By 1988, a review of studies across Canada suggested that edentulism was declining in Ontario but was still very high in Quebec.[59] Indeed, 1985 research found that 78.6 per cent of Quebecers over the age of 65 had full upper dentures, and 65.6 per cent had full lowers. Half of the dentures were judged unsatisfactory. Additionally, 16 per cent of the edentulous lacked dentures or did not wear them. Not surprisingly, tooth retention increased markedly with income. Tellingly, only 42 per cent of Quebecers over 65 perceived themselves as needing oral health care – suggesting how many were willing to put up with poor oral health or regarded it as a normal aspect of aging.[60]

In the 1980s, the dental profession, wrestling with an over-supply of practitioners, finally began to pay more attention to "geriatric dentistry," or gerodontology.[61] In 1982, Irwin Lightman, the dentist at Toronto's Baycrest Centre for Geriatric Care, one of the country's few seniors' homes with a regular dental service, scolded his colleagues in a *JCDA* editorial: "The need for dental care for the elderly of this country is great and we, the dental profession, must address ourselves to this problem now." Studies and surveys were not enough: "We have to go into the nursing homes, old folks homes, chronic hospitals and other extended care facilities, and get to work." Dentists could improve chewing ability and raise self-esteem by replacing missing teeth or constructing dentures. Lightman advised dental schools to begin courses on gerodontology and suggested doing some of the required clinical work on elderly patients.[62] A *JCDA* editorial later that year agreed with Lightman's call to action and announced a conference on "Geriatric Dentistry" at the University of Western Ontario in 1983.[63] In 1984, a *JCDA* editorial suggested that dentists offer seniors a discount of 10–15 per cent to encourage the not-so-well-off to seek care.[64] That same year, a leading Canadian scholar of gerodontology, Michael MacEntee, commented: "The enthusiasm shown by the dental profession for paediatric dentistry has paid off with the control of caries in children and an unprecedented demand for orthodontic treatment from all age groups. Now that children are no longer so demanding of a dentist's time, it is possible for the profession to look towards the grandparents, perhaps to provide this older population with an equally successful service."[65] Even still, progress was slow: few dental schools offered geriatric dentistry.[66] Seniors continued to lack dental care. As I outlined in chapter 3, Alberta was the only province to provide free oral health care to seniors, and at the turn of this century it restricted that to the less affluent.[67] In 1985, Jack Lee, Toronto's dental adviser, revealed that more than half of the city's seniors had not seen a dentist in more than five years – blocked, he suspected, by fear and high cost.[68]

While the rate of tooth loss was declining, elderly Canadians still had very poor oral health. A 1994 study of elderly residents of Collective Living Centres in North York (Toronto) reported that only 30.5 per cent had no teeth. Most of the dentate had more than half of their own teeth. This was a far cry from the situation in the 1970s. Even so, the North Yorkers were in bad shape: many of the dentate required extractions, many dentures needed cleaning or repair, and one-tenth of residents required urgent care because of pain or serious infection.[69] Yet other studies showed dentists little interested in working in such residences: they anticipated minimal demand, inadequate facilities, unsatisfying work, and poor compensation. Younger colleagues and practitioners who had taken courses in geriatric dentistry were more willing.[70]

While tooth loss had declined in prosperous, urban North York, many inequalities remained in the province. The Ontario Health Survey

(1990) showed that people in the north were far more likely to be edentulous than those elsewhere.[71] Poorer people were much more likely to have lost their teeth than the affluent.[72] Highly uneven access to care correlated strongly with dental insurance. The *Canadian Health Measures Survey* 2007–09 revealed that people aged 60–79 were much less likely than other age groups to have dental insurance (53.2 per cent had none). Those uninsured older adults were much less likely to have visited a dentist in the past year (54.5 per cent) than the insured (76.9 per cent).[73] As in other age groups, people with public dental insurance were also significantly less likely to visit a dentist, perhaps because they were unable to find a dentist who would serve them or because they did not see regular dental care as a necessity or feared the pain involved.[74] Indeed, many studies have shown that elderly people often do not consider their oral health problems serious, either out of stoicism or because they have more pressing health issues.[75] This may change as baby boomers, particularly the wealthy ones, demand a higher quality of life as they age.

In the late twentieth century, as the boomers began to reach their 40s and 50s, the age at which many of their parents had lost their teeth, not only had many benefitted from oral health education in their youth and from regular dental care, but recent innovations promised to preserve their teeth, or at least a reasonable facsimile of them. In the early 1990s, after many years of attempts, dental implants became a realistic option for many Canadians, arguably part of the anti-aging medicine that surged in that decade as the boomers reached mid-life.[76] As Carol Haber put it, these folks "came of age in a culture that once defined even those over thirty as old and untrustworthy" so were therefore particularly "invested" in staving off the aging process.[77]

A Canadian, George Zarb, helped introduce effective dental implants. At the University of Toronto, Zarb was working on implants in animal models when he learned about Per-Ingvar Brånemark's work at the University of Gotenborg. Brånemark pioneered implants that seamlessly connected implant and bone (osseointegration). Zarb launched clinical trials of this method in 1979 and organized an influential international conference on the subject in 1982. As a result, the University of Toronto became a world leader in implant therapy.[78] By the early 1990s, implants had become well-accepted, although they were still very expensive and relatively few dentists knew how to perform them. During the decade, many dentists attended special instruction courses.[79] By the early 2000s, implants had become standard in advanced dental practices and were being widely advertised.[80]

A raft of newspaper articles across the country alerted consumers to their advantages.[81] A 2001 article in the *Victoria Times Columnist* (a city with many retirees) raved: "They cost thousands of dollars are made of titanium and can take months to become fully integrated and functional. But people with dental implants almost always wish they'd had them sooner."[82] Brian Lahiffe, a UBC professor of dentistry, enthused, "Implants take people who are social cripples – unable to smile, laugh or even eat in company and turn them into happy vibrant people."[83] Shirley Bouck, a retired nurse, had been hit by a truck as a teenager. It crushed her jaw. She had a variety of bridges and other prostheses, but none of them fitted very well: "I used to have face aches, headaches. You can't imagine it unless you've had teeth wobbling around in your head. It was terrible. My implants cost about $13,000 but there is nothing like having good teeth. They're a blessing."[84] According to the *Windsor Star*, eighty-year-old Jake Hunter had only five teeth and a badly fitting lower denture when he decided to spend $20,000 on implants, saying: "I'll socialize more once I have the teeth. It was too difficult to eat out before."[85] After his surgery, he boasted that he was going home to have steak.

That said, dental implants and other forms of dental prostheses are not perfect. As one systemic review concluded: "Despite the high survival of FDP[s] [fixed dental prostheses] biological and technical complications were frequent. This, in turn, means that substantial amounts of chair time have to be accepted by the patient, by dental services and by society at large following the incorporation of FDPs."[86] Manufacturers have heavily marketed implants, many of which had little testing.[87] The devices remain very costly – as Michael MacEntee explained in a 1999 instruction manual, "Poor people are in no position to seek the benefits of dental implants."[88] Finally, a small literature suggests that not everyone wants to become "a cyborg" with replacement parts – for some people, these new technologies, which also include hip and knee replacements and pacemakers, feel unnatural, or work less well than the organs they were intended to replace.[89]

The implant revolution was part of the transition to cosmetic dentistry. As oral health has improved, dentistry shifted from "need-based" to "want-based." As an article in a journal of dental-practice management outlined in 2004, "If you've made your living on need-based dentistry, we hope you're ready to retire because 90 per cent of the future financial growth in the industry will be in want-based dentistry."[90] Cosmetic dentistry, of course, is not about just implants: it also includes veneers, whitening, and other interventions that can make teeth look better and patients younger. But implants were far from just cosmetic: for some people they significantly improved their quality of life.

Conclusion

In the mid-twentieth century, denturists and their supporters fought a hard battle for recognition as health professionals. They succeeded partly because of the great need for cost-effective dentures. But by the early 2000s, people were keeping their teeth for much longer. Many who lost teeth were able to replace them with implants. There is something to celebrate here: dentures are not a satisfactory replacement for natural teeth. Yet keeping one's teeth required substantial work and expense. For most people, it meant daily oral hygiene and regular visits to a dentist. Also, these benefits have been uneven: people in long-term-care homes might have more of their teeth, but still suffer disproportionately from poor oral health. People living in poverty do not have access to these new interventions. The Non-Insured Health Benefits Program, which provides dental insurance to registered First Nations members and Inuit in Canada, notably does not provide dental implants.[91] As the majority of Canadians improve their oral health, missing teeth, bad breath, or even stained teeth become even more of an employment or social liability than they were 50 years ago. The privatized nature of dentistry has discouraged practitioners from treating underserved populations. Many of us are keeping our teeth for a lifetime, but this advance has worsened earlier inequalities in oral health.

6

Hollywood Smiles

The Rise of Cosmetic Dentistry

In 1976, *Charlie Angels* actress Farrah Fawcett (figure 6.1) became a pin-up star with her dazzling, almost incandescent smile. The famous photo (reportedly the best-selling poster of all time) of her in her red bathing suit had her baring both her upper and lower teeth, all of them blindingly white.[1] While her famous hair received even more praise than her teeth, her grin helped set the stage for what smiles could look like and ushered in an era of almost impossibly large smiles set with exceedingly straight and even teeth. By the turn of the century, cosmetic dentistry was so pervasive in Hollywood that *Globe and Mail* movie critic Johanna Schneller reported that "tooth mania has taken over the multiplex. Look at that searing examination of dental care in small-town America that opened last week, *Teaching Mrs. Jingle*. Nominally, it is about three high school seniors who tie their evil history teacher to her bed. For me, however, it's about how every person in the town – including the teacher (Helen Mirren), the smartest student (Katie Holmes) and her down and out name-tag wearing waitress mom (Lesley Ann Warren) has flawless, radiantly white teeth." She noted that Matt Damon's "Olympic-calibre choppers" in *Good Will Hunting* "made working-class South Boston look like the dental care capital of the world."[2]

By the 1980s, the oral health of the Canadian population had drastically improved, and many people had employer-provided dental benefits that covered much of the medically necessary care. The shortage of dentists had eased, especially in large cities, where practitioners, especially new ones, lacked patients. Middle-class baby boomers, many of whom had benefitted from fluorides in their youth, were beginning to believe that they, unlike most of their parents, might keep their teeth for life and were more willing to invest in them. New materials allowed dentists to do more – reshape mouths and teeth to create the perfect

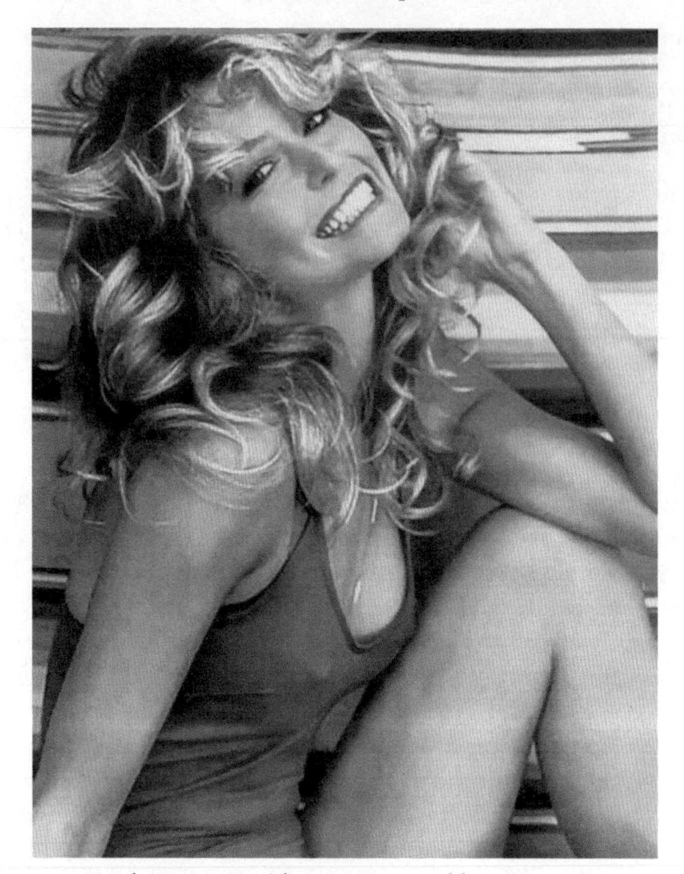

6.1 Farah Fawcett's wide grin (captured here in 1976) helped set new standards for smiles.

smile. The wide smiles of movie stars and celebrities made some people long for the same. By the early 2000s, "makeover" shows on television gave consumers a vivid picture of what dentists could accomplish.

As a result, "aesthetic" or "cosmetic dentistry" exploded. Some adults were wearing braces, tooth whitening became a craze, and some invested in more extreme procedures like porcelain veneers and gum reshaping. While the health aspect of dentistry never disappeared, more practitioners focused on the cosmetic nature of their practice. In the meantime, some Canadians started to have new expectations for what their smiles should look like – for some, this meant undergoing painful, expensive, and time-consuming procedures in the name of beauty. This trend ultimately exacerbated class inequalities – only wealthier people could afford the new treatments – while also establishing new norms for what the smile should look like. Smiles that were once fully acceptable were becoming a liability in the workplace and might now hold one back on the job or in the quest for love. It is also noticeable that the majority of cosmetic dentistry is done on women, showing that women still face much higher expectations in terms of personal appearance than men, and many women seem far more willing to submit to pain, expense, and risk to achieve an idealized form.[3]

Orthodontics

The transition to cosmetic dentistry began with orthodontics. Although humans have tried as far back as ancient Egypt to move teeth, the modern specialty of orthodontics emerged in the United States in the late nineteenth century.[4] Its so-called father was Dr Edward Angle (1855–1930), who wrote classic works on orthodontic practices and was the first to classify malocclusions – misalignments between the teeth when the jaws are closed. Angle created his own school of orthodontia in St Louis, Missouri, in 1899 and trained many of the field's first practitioners.[5] Historian Elizabeth Hunt contends that it was orthodontists, especially Angle, who created the "standard bite" by classifying malocclusions.[6] These classifications changed over time, but implied that many people needed their teeth fixed to meet these norms. While severe malocclusions can lead to oral health problems, measuring bites was more about standardizing appearance than about medical need. Indeed, various systems assessed orthodontic need differently: between 1930 and 1965 in the United States, the proportion of misaligned mouths varied in studies from 35 per cent to 95 per cent.[7]

US orthodontics grew rapidly after 1900, when the American Society of Orthodontists was established. By the 1930s, there were two academic journals in the field, and by 1945, eighteen university dental schools were offering courses.[8] In Canada, growth was slower, reflecting the smaller dental profession and the corresponding lack of educational opportunities. In 1947, Canada had 40 orthodontists all in major urban centres – 13 in Montreal, 12 in Toronto, 3 in Winnipeg, 2 in Ottawa, and 1 each in Vancouver, Victoria, Windsor, and Hamilton – and one place offering training: the Université de Montréal.[9] Most first-generation practitioners trained in the United States, and the field would maintain close cross-border intellectual ties: even when Canadian dental schools started offering graduate courses in orthodontics, many of the professors were American, as were the textbooks and journals. In short, even after Canada opened more programs, students were exposed to the same textbooks and literature as Americans, and practice norms and philosophies were very similar.

In Canada, orthodontics expanded quickly following the Second World War, especially in the more populous and wealthier provinces. By 1961, there were 116 practitioners in the country: 61 in Ontario, 26 in Quebec, 9 in British Columbia, and 8 in Alberta. Prince Edward Island and Newfoundland had none, and there were only a handful elsewhere. By 1984, the country had a total of 475: half in Ontario, and a disproportionate number in the wealthier provinces of British Columbia and Alberta.[10]

The growth in the field corresponded with cultural changes emphasizing appearance. Kathy Peiss, Elizabeth Haiken, and Jane Nicholas have argued that the popularity of visual culture in North America in the 1920s and 1930s, including magazines and movies, made people, especially women, more conscious of how they looked and created new expectations for women's bodies and faces.[11] While few scholars have examined teeth as an element of this change, the widespread use of porcelain veneers for teeth in Hollywood and the interwar explosion of toothpaste advertising (see chapter 1), helped create a cultural preference for gleaming white smiles with straight, even teeth.[12] In his history of smiling, Fred Schroeder argues that it was not until the interwar years that smiling became a positive form of self-presentation for everyone – previously it was intended to portray people who were lower class or evil. Dale Carnegie's 1936 bestseller, *How to Win Friends and Influence People*, counselled readers that smiling was a superb way to get people to like them.[13]

As Melissa Micu and I have explored elsewhere, orthodontists argued that their work could cure "inferiority complexes." In *Applied Orthodontia* (which would be released in seven editions from 1922 to 1956), James McCoy highlighted his field's benefits: better chewing, breathing, and facial harmony, but also healthier, happier children: "Personality is perhaps the greatest factor in life ... A child with a receding chin, protruding upper teeth and short, under-developed upper lip is often judged weak or stupid because of its appearance." Such a youngster often develops "traits of indecision and weakness." Similarly, those with protruding mandibles (lower jawbones) were often thought pugnacious, whatever their character. Crooked or misaligned teeth could prevent the "self-poise and self-confidence which are so essential to success and happiness in later life." McCoy promised that orthodontics could imprint on a child's face "a personality which is the true expression of its character."[14]

George Anderson's much-used *Practical Orthodontics* (1948) pronounced that "esthetic disharmony" frequently causes "a mental complex," because of teasing or unkind comments. "True personality may be hidden, or even a false personality created." Anderson promised that orthodontic treatment can "give many of these afflicted individuals a new and far more pleasant outlook on life." It could also improve a child's chewing, reduce gum disease, and remedy speech defects, but tellingly, the writer placed psychological concerns first.[15] T.M. Graber's classic text *Orthodontics: Principles and Practice* (1961) concluded: "The psychological implications of a severe malocclusion can be enormous. Many an adult neurosis or impotent or misdirected motivational drive can be traced to childhood attitudes begot by the cruel intolerance of a face-conscious society."[16]

The psychological justification for orthodontic treatment was echoed in the popular press. In 1948, an article in *Maclean's* magazine promoted the wonders of orthodontics. It featured a little boy, Johnnie, who was nicknamed "Tusky" when he started school because of his protruding upper teeth and so "was never one of the boys." His front teeth did not meet when his mouth was closed, so he needed to cut his food into small pieces to eat it. He could not eat apples or sandwiches like other children. Continuously teased, he became both an outcast and a bully with a severe "inferiority complex." At age ten, he had already been convicted of petty theft. That same year, a group of older boys beat him up, loosening his four upper front teeth. His mother took him for the first time to the dentist, who referred her to an orthodontist. After that, Johnnie wore braces for a year. His teeth realigned, and the look of his face improved. At the time of writing, he was "the most popular junior rugby halfback in his city and a good looking six-footer to boot."[17] The article, like many others in the period, argued that crooked teeth could warp a child's personality and development and that fixing them could be transformative. In 1957, the Canadian Dental Association sponsored the National Film Board's *Putting It Straight: A Story of Crooked Teeth*, in which Mary's whole personality was distorted by her crooked teeth.[18]

It is not surprising that this film focused on a girl: the limited evidence suggests that parents were more likely to treat girls' malocclusions than boys'. In 1963, Toronto orthodontist R.O. Fisk reported that 56.5 per cent of the children in his practice were female; he concluded that parents were more likely to think that less-serious malocclusions were not as important in boys as they were in girls.[19] In 1976, 36 per cent of twelve-year-olds in Forest Hill Village (a wealthy community in Toronto, well-served by orthodontists) were receiving treatment – 60 per cent of them were female.[20] Some parents saw fixing a girl's teeth as helping her to prepare for adulthood, including marriage. As an article in *Saturday Night* revealed: "A little girl of four may have scarcely noticeable protruding teeth. No one worries about it. But when that girl is eighteen her heart may be breaking because of her unsightly teeth."[21] Indeed, the preponderance of female patients had one Toronto paediatric dentist railing against the "old fogey" notion that "only girls should be given expensive orthodontic treatment. There's no such thing as girl and boy dentistry. Boys should get the same treatment as girls."[22] Indeed, as numerous historians and feminist scholars have shown, expectations were much higher for women's appearance than for men's, making adolescent girls much more anxious over their looks than teenage boys.[23] Girls also faced much greater pressure to smile. While smiling in North America has long been a way of putting other people at ease and creating connection, it is often a gendered responsibility, with women – especially those of lower status – needing to appear friendly and unthreatening.[24] Thus it was not at all unusual that parents were more likely to repair their daughter's teeth than their son's.

In the 1970s, the idea that crooked teeth caused insoluble psychological problems was called into question by several studies that showed that malocclusion did not have a significant impact on people's psychological health.[25] Even so, orthodontists, such as William R. Profitt, who wrote the field's best-selling textbook in the 1980s, argued that research had confirmed "what is intuitively obvious, that severe malocclusion can be a social handicap" and "well-aligned teeth and a pleasing smile" socially advantageous. He claimed that teachers, prospective marriage partners, and employers all valued appearance. At the same time, he recognized the inequalities: wealthy youngsters had more orthodontic treatment than the poor, and girls more than boys.[26]

Meanwhile the number of orthodontists in Canada skyrocketed. In 2001, there were 666 licensed orthodontists.[27] By this time, the cohort of pre-teens and teenagers (the most likely subjects) was shrinking. Moreover, dentists anxious about declining patient rolls began doing orthodontics too, increasing competition.[28] In response, orthodontists intensified their marketing. In the early 1980s, the Canadian Association of Orthodontists ran several advertisements in *Chatelaine*, Canada's leading women's magazine. The first featured a smiling, red-headed, freckled girl with a pronounced gap between her front teeth; another tooth was chipped. The ad suggested that her smile had personality but that the "cute smile" might be hiding "teeth she may not be able to live with." It promised that treatment could improve appearance and "mouth health."[29] Another ad, two years later, featured a smiling mother and child, but warned, "They're showing you a potentially serious health problem" despite their "very acceptable smiles."[30] Orthodontists apparently took an equally heavy hand in their offices. One mother, who had been to several offices in search of the right treatment for her children, told the *Toronto Star* that some "play on your feelings. They say, 'you don't want your kid to grow up with ugly teeth, they'll never smile.'"[31] One orthodontist interviewed for the same article proclaimed: "It is 'absolutely clear' that in our culture people with straight teeth feel better about themselves … People equate straight teeth with wealth, happiness and success. Parents should recognize that this is a very significant factor with a huge impact."[32] Dr Arlene Dagys, a past president of the Ontario Association of Orthodontists, seconded this, "No one ever died of crooked teeth … But the psychological benefits are very important."[33] As early as 1981, one Calgary practitioner was claiming that 35 per cent of his patients were adults, compared to just 2–3 per cent five years earlier.[34] By 1986, the Canadian Association of Orthodontists estimated that 25 per cent of patients were adults.[35] Probably even more of these were female than among child patients. Dr Ray Bozek, head of the Ontario Society of Orthodontists, noted that adult women often outnumbered adult male patients by two to one.[36] In 1991, *La Presse* in Montreal claimed that adults received almost 40 per cent of orthodontic treatment, with two-thirds of them women, mostly in their late twenties.[37]

There were numerous reasons for this increase. Many patients whose parents had not been able to afford treatment for them were now able to pay for it themselves. As adult work became more common, it became more socially acceptable to sport tinsel teeth.[38] As well, attitudes towards teeth were changing. Until the 1980s, rates of adult tooth loss remained high, and many people expected to wear dentures. But baby boomers were more likely to preserve their teeth, increasing their motivation for orthodontic work.[39] The growth in adult orthodontics made it more socially acceptable to admit that such treatment was primarily for aesthetic reasons. Despite the improvements in orthodontic treatment, it remains painful and embarrassing for many teenagers, as Raina Telgemeier's best-selling graphic novel *Smile*, about her own experiences in the 1980s, makes acutely clear.[40] Parents perhaps loath to subject their children to the pain of orthodontic treatment or worried about the hefty costs wanted to believe at least that treatment would give their offspring improved mental health and increase their chances of happiness. Adults, who assumed the embarrassment and pain for themselves, could more easily think of it as self-improvement.

The surge in adult orthodontics might reflect also technological advances of the 1970s and 1980s. The heavy metal braces and headgear of the 1950s and 1960s were less common. New devices, such as lingual braces, placed on the backside of the teeth, eased adult treatment.[41] Innovative materials, such as spring clips, ceramics, and better bonding agents, made braces less noticeable and more efficient, straightening teeth sooner. By 2000, coloured wires and elastics had some orthodontists claiming that children were disappointed not to need braces.[42] Also in the 1980s and 1990s, new digital technologies were employed that allowed patients to visualize how treatment could transform their face. Ms Challis, thirty-six years old, told a journalist that she immediately liked a computer-generated image of her post-treatment face: "I wasn't an ugly duckling before or anything, but the picture with my lower jaw brought forward was really great, it really fixed up my chin."[43] By the early 2000s, products like Invisalign, clear plastic trays worn over the teeth to move them gradually into shape, had taken the market by storm.[44]

Whitening, Gum Contouring, and Veneers

Adult orthodontics was the most time-consuming procedure for patients, but there was no shortage of other interventions to improve the look of their teeth. The most common was whitening. Teeth darken naturally with age, giving them a yellow appearance. In the 1990s, bleaching became common at many dental offices. For professional whitening, dentists would provide a custom mouth guard. Patients would apply whitening gel at home and keep the guard on for 2–8 hours per day for two weeks. The process cost about $600–$1,000.[45] At the turn of the century, many dentists began offering laser whitening, which used heat to make the peroxide more effective.[46] As well, over-the-counter products proliferated.[47] In *Chatelaine* in the 2000s, virtually all the oral hygiene ads were for Crest Whitestrips and whitening toothpastes.[48]

These new technologies reshaped many people's standards for white teeth. Toronto dentist Dana Colson told the *Globe and Mail* that "they've had to totally redesign the charts" as patients' perception of what it meant to have white teeth changed.[49] Many patients sought to match their teeth with the whites of the eyes.[50] As Leslie Faust, the CEO of GoSmile, which made teeth-whitening products, informed the *Edmonton Journal* in 2008: "These days there's almost no such thing as too white."[51] Many dentists began offering free whitening to lure new patients.[52] Celebrities took up the procedure with alacrity. According to Sylvie Vallières of the Ordre des dentistes du Québec, "Almost every Quebec artist has had their teeth whitened. Programs on TV, like *Extreme Makeover*, are having an effect. More people are asking for more information about whitening, bridges and orthodontics."[53]

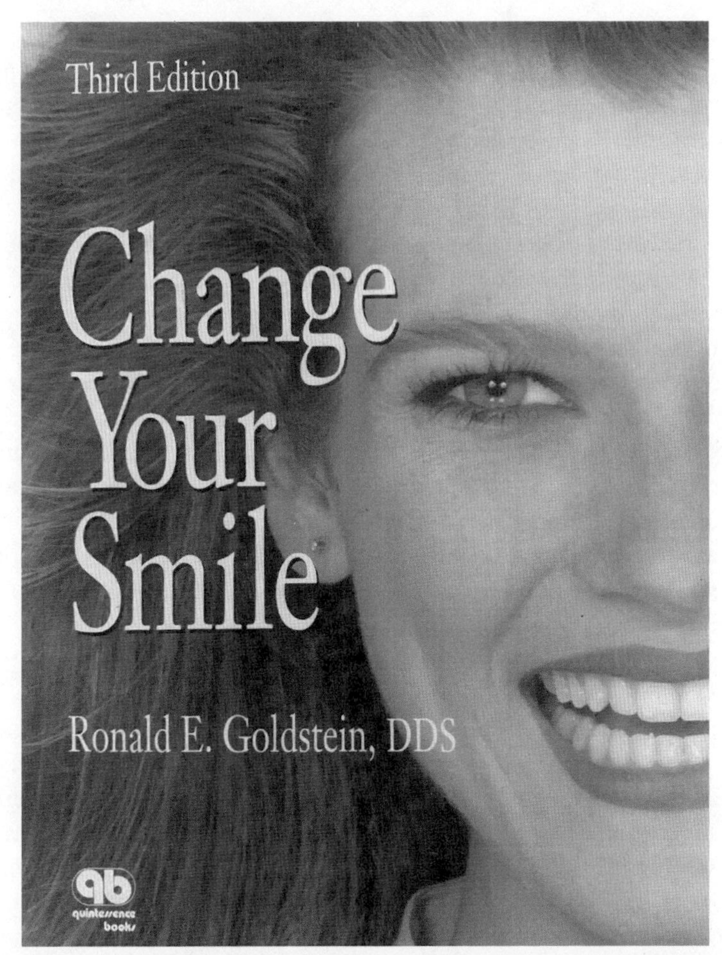

6.2 Ronald Goldstein's *Change Your Smile* (3rd ed., 1996) showed patients how dentists could transform their smiles.

Another way to obtain white, even teeth, was by applying veneers. Porcelain veneers were first made in the 1920s for Hollywood stars by Charles Pincus.[54] But these often became loose because of primitive bonding agents and techniques. Porcelain veneers could cover stained, chipped, or uneven teeth, even conceal gaps. *Change Your Smile* (figure 6.2), a text written by leading cosmetic dentist Ronald Goldstein for patients, described how he used veneers to cover the teeth of a thirteen-year-old after they had been badly stained by the antibiotic tetracycline. Boys had started calling her names because of her teeth, and he warned that "unless attention is paid to esthetic problems of young people, severe personality problems may develop." This, of course, was very similar to the language promoting orthodontics. The before and after photos contrasted her small, stained teeth with a beautiful piano-key-white smile. Goldstein concluded: "Notice how much more beautiful she looks after the bonding. It is easy to understand how one's self-confidence can be enhanced following a cosmetic improvement."[55] Acrylic veneers were another option: these did not last as long as porcelain veneers or provide the same tooth-like translucency, but they were quicker, less expensive, and less damaging to the original tooth material.[56] Another procedure was gum surgery to remove excessive gum tissue. Goldstein described one patient, a twenty-year-old Miss America contestant who showed too much gum when she smiled. He made her teeth look longer by removing some of her gum tissue. Afterwards he reported, "Her teeth appear longer and much less gum tissue shows when she smiles, which gave her much more self-confidence."[57] Dentists could also fix chipped teeth, reshape teeth to make them look more "feminine" or more "masculine," increase the size of small teeth, and change the look of the lips.[58]

Why Have Cosmetic Dentistry?

The decision to have cosmetic dentistry had much in common with the rationale for plastic surgery. Cosmetic dentists (and many patients) raved about its impact on confidence and self-esteem. Montreal dentist Dr George Freeman enthused in 1986 that veneers "often increases a person's self-confidence because they no longer worry about the appearance of their teeth." He added: "A nice smile can be the high point of a face."[59] Dr Charles Kamel of Ottawa reported: "Esthetic dentistry is a very emotional form of dentistry. You can change someone's self-perception in as short a time as one appointment. It creates confidence, gives people a different outlook on themselves, and therefore, a greater possibility of success."[60] Dr Gordon Chee of Calgary's Aesthetic Dental Studio considered his practice "most rewarding in terms of improving patients' self-esteem and self-confidence." It seemed to him inseparable from medical care: "Sometimes, people's teeth are quite damaged because of bite problems, chipped teeth and so on. So you deal with their dental health first, then the appearance later to ensure the longevity of what you are putting in their mouths. That way, you really make a difference to people's lives."[61]

Patients also praised the effects. In 1987, Barbara Atchie, a businesswoman in her early thirties, said that she had veneers put on because in business she always noticed other people's teeth. "I'm pleased that now I can smile and my teeth may not be perfect-looking but will just look like good teeth." Charles Lapointe, a business consultant, also in his thirties, had his teeth capped so they would no longer look crooked: "With the work that I've had done, I think my smile is a lot softer and more appealing."[62] Karen Wilson, a dog groomer in her twenties, reported that before her porcelain veneers and gingivectomy she used to cover her mouth when meeting new people. Men could tell that she didn't feel good about herself. Since her procedures, she told the *Toronto Star*, "I can talk with people; I'm happier. And I smile a lot. People say that I'm more confident."[63]

Growth of Cosmetic Dentistry

Cosmetic dentistry grew rapidly in the last quarter of the twentieth century. The American Academy of Esthetic Dentistry was founded in 1975, followed in 1984 by the American Academy for Cosmetic Surgery.[64] The Toronto Academy for Cosmetic Dentistry was set up in 1987 with 20 members; by 1995, it had 150.[65] The Canadian Academy of Aesthetic Dentistry was created in 2004.[66] The first major textbook, Ronald Goldstein's *Esthetics in Dentistry*, came out in 1976. The *Journal of Esthetic and Restorative Dentistry*, the first in the field, emerged in 1998. The *Journal of the Canadian Dental Association* (JCDA) devoted its first issue to cosmetic dentistry in April 1988. (Ironically, April was National Dental Health Month.) Its theme that year was "Keep Smiling" – perhaps an indication of the growing enthusiasm for cosmetic dentistry within the profession. Previous themes had been more health-oriented, such as 1986's "Support Your Teeth" and 1985's "Dental Health: Good for Life."[67] The journal reprinted an editorial from the *Journal of the American Dental Association* suggesting that in the past, dentistry had been concerned primarily with alleviating pain and preventing disease, but recently "tremendous technological advances" had "allowed patients to expect and to receive the very best in esthetic dental treatments from their dentists." The introduction of fluorides had created a generation of caries-free children – an opportunity "to enter the real golden age of dentistry, taking a new direction with esthetic dentistry as its banner."[68]

In the mid-1990s, with dental insurance being cut back and oral health continuing to improve, dentists looked to uninsured, elective procedures to keep their practices profitable.[69] Their educational outreach focused on increasing their elective or cosmetic work.[70] In 1994, the Ontario Dental Association launched a campaign for cosmetic dentistry. One billboard showed the word "GAP" with a large space between the G and the A: "Fixing it is easier than you think."[71] In 2000, the Université de Montréal added cosmetic dentistry and implants to its curriculum.[72] In 2001, a survey of sixty-four North American dental schools found that roughly half had a course on cosmetic dentistry, in place on average for three years. The other half reported that a variety of courses included the subject, while 15 per cent were developing a course. Of the schools that had a course, most (92 per cent) included aesthetic assessments in diagnosis and treatment planning.[73]

The first "cosmetic dentists" opened in wealthy shopping districts like Toronto's Yorkville, rife with high-end boutiques, or in the tony suburbs of West Vancouver.[74] By the early 2000s, dentists in communities like Cranbrook, British Columbia; Regina, Saskatchewan; and St Catharines, Ontario, were doing cosmetic procedures.[75] The field's expansion was aided by the Supreme Court of Canada's decision in 1990 that allowed dentists to advertise their services. In 1985, Toronto dentist Howard Rocket and his business partner, dentist Brian Price, who were trailblazers in "retail dentistry," were featured in a series of ads in *Canadian Business*, the *Financial Post*, the *Financial Times*, *Maclean's*, *Newsweek*, and *Time*. The campaign was paid for by Holiday Inn, which was promoting these dentists' stays at the hotel during business travel. The ads positioned them as "visionaries" who had opened seventy new offices in a short time. By this point, their company, Tridont, was North America's largest storefront-dentistry operation.[76] The Royal College of Dental Surgeons of Ontario launched disciplinary proceedings against Rocket and Price for advertising. The dentists retorted that the regulation was an unconstitutional violation of their right to free speech. After a decision in their favour by a lower court, the Supreme Court concurred in [1990] 2 SCR 232.[77]

By 2000, over half of advertising dentists in Toronto promoted cosmetic dentistry.[78] By 2005, some dentists had full-page ads in the *Yellow Pages* featuring individuals, couples, and families with broad smiles.[79] Couples were particularly common, reflecting the growing romantic value of straight, white teeth. Indeed, even before advertising became legal, dentists were reporting spillover from the United States, where the American Dental Association had removed its restrictions in 1979.[80] Patients in Canada were requesting enamel bonding, which was being pushed extensively on US cable TV.[81]

The growing glut of dentists in big cities spurred the drive towards cosmetic dentistry. Donald Lewis's 1981 study of dental personnel in Ontario revealed that 32 per cent of general practitioners were less busy than they would like to be, as were nearly half of the 1970–78 graduates.[82] The ratio of dentists to people kept increasing: by 1992, there was one dentist for every 1,919 Canadians.[83] Two decades earlier, when dental needs on average were much greater there was one dentist for every 2,749.[84] As journalist Jan Wong asserted in 1996: "Dentists are bleeding. Three decades of fluoridated water and toothpaste, a glut of graduates and a nineties erosion of welfare and corporate benefits have taken a big bite out of the profession."[85] According to Dr Edward Philips, a former member of the executive of the Ontario Dental Association, in 1995 a dozen dentists went bankrupt, compared to none through the entire 1980s. Banks were becoming reluctant to lend money to dentists.[86]

In response to the perceived over-supply, in 1983 and 1984 the two Ontario dental schools (Toronto and Western) cut enrolment by 21 per cent. In 1987, Dalhousie also shrank its incoming dental class. The Professional Resource Utilization Committee of the Canadian Dental Association agreed that dental faculties needed to examine enrolment numbers. Toronto decreased its freshman class from 128 to 104 in 1987 and to 80 in 1988. McGill also made cuts.[87] Many universities considered shuttering their dental school. McGill's nearly closed in the early 1990s, saved by private funds, while part-time instructors took a pay cut and several professors retired early.[88] In 1994, Martha Piper, vice-president of research and external affairs at Alberta, proposed closing its school of dentistry.[89] At Saskatchewan, the President's Committee on Renewal suggested looking at ending its program.[90]

While closing schools might have lessened supply, the problem was more complicated. If more Canadians went to the dentist regularly, more dentists would be required. One solution to the expense of running a dental program further fed the growth of cosmetic dentistry. Tuition fees for dental students shot up at the turn of the century, as many provinces deregulated fees. For example, at Saskatchewan, a dental student paid $600 per year in 1970 (or $4,006 in 2019 dollars), $1,985 in 1990 (or $3,431 in 2019 dollars), but $32,960 in 2010 (or $38,402 in 2019 dollars).[91] At Toronto, a dentistry student coughed up $454 in 1951 (or $4,385 in 2019 dollars),[92] $1,100 in 1971 (or $7,100 in 2019 dollars),[93] but $14,000 in 2001 ($19,339 in 2019 dollars).[94] As a result, dental students were graduating with increasingly large debts, meaning that establishing a viable practice was top-of-mind for young graduates. One route: set up a practice that provided cosmetic work in addition to fillings, root canals, and cleanings.

In the 1980s and 1990s, as their debts increased and competition for patients intensified, dentists spent more time thinking about practice management. A 1988 article in the JCDA suggested that Goldstein's *Change Your Smile* should be in the reception room of every dental office.[95] A regular columnist for the JCDA, Imtiaz Manji, a principal of Exper-Dent Consultants, argued that, with patients disappearing, dentists needed to promote treatment plans – long-term plans for dental work in their mouths. He argued that the time was ripe because of "increasing patient demand for esthetic procedures, as well as new treatment modalities such as implants." He argued that profits could increase by 30 per cent if offices could talk patients into treatment plans.[96] Such recommendations were often cosmetic. One easy way to generate business was through persuading patients that their silver-amalgam fillings should be replaced with tooth-coloured composites, for either health or aesthetic reasons. In December 1990, *60 Minutes* on CBS TV did a program on mercury fillings, suggesting that they might be the cause of numerous diseases, including Alzheimer's, arthritis, and colitis.[97] It featured Calgary dentist Murray Vimy, who claimed that amalgam fillings regularly released mercury vapour.[98] Vimy eventually published a book called *Your Toxic Teeth*.[99] While most evidence suggests that these substances are safe (and last longer than composites), many patients and dentists decided to err on the side of caution and have them removed.[100]

The gurus of cosmetic dentistry had numerous suggestions for increasing business. Goldstein suggested asking every patient to fill out a "Smile Analysis" after the first visit. Twenty questions probed the colour, length, evenness, and proportion of the patient's teeth, the appearance of their gums, the smell of their breath. Goldstein suggested that the questionnaire provided a way for the dentist to avoid a "common error" of thinking that the patient was not interested in aesthetic treatment, but obviously it could also be used to create the desire for aesthetic treatment by persuading a patient that there was something wrong with their smile.[101] A similar checklist appeared in Kenneth Aschheim and Barry G. Dale's text *Esthetic Dentistry* (2001). Various types of similar surveys became common in dental practices across North America.[102]

The second edition of Goldstein's *Esthetics in Dentistry* (1998) added a chapter on marketing and strongly recommended displaying a book like *Change Your Smile* extolling the wonders of cosmetic dentistry.[103] The marketing chapter warned that patients looking for discounts might not be worth the trouble.[104] While the text suggested a "neat and attractive" office, the photos showed luxurious art, furniture, and fresh flowers.[105] Such spaces, which have proliferated, can create obstacles to care in that many patients do not feel comfortable in such posh surroundings. Research has shown that people with lower incomes prefer a public clinic or dental school to a private office.[106]

Indeed, cosmetic dentistry rose in tandem with "spa dentistry." In about 2000, some dentists started offering patients noise-cancelling headphones and TVs, aromatherapy, massage, and even Botox. At Spa Dentaire Laurier in Montreal, a therapist massaged patient's hands and feet during the treatment. Dentist Pierre Comeau said: "I wanted to create an environment that was better for me and my patients. I have taken a Zen approach with colours and aromas to make patients more comfortable and relaxed. This put patients in a better mood. It helps in the healing process." He reported that his patients were mostly in their twenties and thirties and two-thirds were female. More than 60 per cent of his business was in cosmetic dentistry.[107] In Toronto, dentist Sol Weiss's Art of Dentistry offered aromatherapy alongside treatments.[108] A few years later, he opened a practice with a doctor who could expand lips and remove wrinkles with products such as Artecoll, Botox, and Retylane.[109] In Elliot Mechanic's dental office in Montreal, patients could watch films with virtual-reality glasses, have their hands treated with paraffin, and receive aromatherapy. He said, "*Je ne veux plus que les gens considèrent la visite chez le dentiste comme une expérience douloureuse ou pénible. Je ne veux plus qu'ils aient peur de venir.*"[110] In Vancouver, A Smile Above Design Inc. in Coal Harbour offered cosmetic dentistry along with Botox and other facial rejuvenations.[111]

Cosmetic dentistry received a boost from the growing popularity of cosmetic surgery. In *Reshaping the Female Body*, Kathy Davis reveals that magazines started to publish articles on cosmetic surgery in the late 1960s and early 1970s. After 1975, profiles abounded in mainstream magazines. Davis argues that the magazines presented surgery "as a relatively harmless way to improve appearance – an acceptable path towards happiness and well-being."[112] While Statistics Canada does not collect data on people undertaking plastic surgery, the number of board-certified plastic surgeons increased from just over 400 in 1995 to well over 600 in 2018.[113] Since a physician does not need certification to do "cosmetic" surgery, it undoubtedly expanded much more. US cosmetic procedures nearly doubled from 1997 to 2003.[114]

TV programs like *Extreme Makeover* (ABC, 2002–07) and *The Swan* (Fox, 2004) helped to popularize cosmetic dentistry, as both had cosmetic dentists on the transformation team. Both shows were extremely popular – *Extreme Makeover* was eventually eclipsed by *Extreme Makeover: Home Edition*, but in its first season attracted more than ten million viewers. *The Swan*, far more exploitative, was cancelled after two seasons, but reportedly attracted large audiences in the first.[115] *Extreme Makeover* usually featured working-class white women, who often had terrible dental problems.[116] In one episode, dentist Bill Dorfman worked on New Jersey resident Kimberly Rodriguez, who had badly damaged and decayed teeth, with the front ones severely protruding. She complained that she never smiled, and that the repair was not about "vanity" but a "necessity." Most viewers would have agreed. Her reaction to her new teeth was heart-warming. Dorfman comes across as warm and caring, though with a somewhat-alarming tendency to hug his patients. The reconstruction is described in great detail –"Extraction of six front teeth, gum and lip repositioning, upper and lower ridges for ten teeth, Galaxy dentures, root canal and five da Vinci veneers" – allowing viewers to make similar requests. As dentist Tom Hedge wrote in *Dental Economics*, Dorfman came across as a "hero," as everyone grasped that "the dental part of the makeover was, perhaps, the most significant."[117] The writer of a book on marketing for dentists first saw *Extreme Makeover* with a class of dentists who considered the show "the greatest thing that ever happened for dentistry's public relations." In his view, its popularity "changed the way the public viewed dentistry and changed the way dentists viewed themselves. Overnight, we wanted to do more cosmetic procedures."[118]

In Britain, a detailed semiotic analysis of a similar makeover show, *Embarrassing Bodies*, concluded that it positioned cosmetic dentistry as solving oral health problems, downplayed patients' knowledge and consent, and portrayed "aesthetic appearance as being the entirety of oral health, not just an important aspect of it."[119] While we cannot do the same analysis for *Extreme Makeover* or *The Swan*, as full editions no longer exist, the remaining clips on YouTube suggest that they prioritized aesthetics over oral health and that the smiles they created were nearly identical.[120]

Ethics of Cosmetic Dentistry

Not all dentists felt comfortable with the transition to cosmetic work. Some worried that it would harm the profession's status. A member of the editorial board of the *Journal of the American Dental Association*, Gordon Christensen, suspected that dentists were falling on the list of the most trusted professions. He believed that "aggressive treatment planning" and the extension into many elective areas had "caused a change in the public's confidence." He urged his colleagues to carefully distinguish for patients which procedures were essential for the "preservation of their oral or systemic health" and which were elective.[121] The dean of the College of Dental Medicine at Midwestern University in Illinois, Richard J. Simonsen, complained: "The code of primum non nocere – first and foremost do no harm – seems to have been cast aside in the headlong pursuit of outrageous overtreatment for financial gain by some."[122] He believed that patients were being pressed into treatments that would not last and would require ongoing care. Many dentists worried about unintended harms – a 2010 article in the *British*

Dental Journal argued that porcelain-laminate veneers (PLVS) made sense for heavily restored teeth with defective restorations, but not to change the colour of the teeth. PLVS could lead to "possible pulpal damage, infection, fractures or even tooth loss" and were equivalent to "amputation and mutilation."[123] Dentist Donald Mulcahy foresaw cosmetic dentistry leading to "over-treatment by exploiting human vanity and ignorance of dentistry, and its less costly, more biologically acceptable alternatives." The accompanying "aggressive, overzealous business attitude" might "diminish our significance as a true health profession."[124] Arthur Schafer, an ethicist at the University of Manitoba, commented that "the increasingly prominent role of cosmetic dentistry poses a potentially serious threat to the moral integrity of the dental profession. The danger is that dentists, for reasons more to do with economics than devotion to their patients' interest, may find themselves selling their cosmetic services in an unprofessional manner."[125]

Some commentators suggested that cosmetic dentists should no longer consider themselves dentists. Jos V.M. Welie, a specialist in health-care ethics, argues that while cosmetic dentists took the view that their procedures were medically necessary in terms of the World Health Organization's definition of health as a state of complete physical, mental, and social well-being, this meant that a $100,000 smile was the ethical equivalent of a $100,000 kidney transplant. In his view, this absurd example showed that "the line of argumentation must have gone wrong." He concluded: "Most cosmetic interventions do not qualify as medical treatment proper because they do not restore a patient's health." He maintained that cosmetic dentists were not medical professionals, although perhaps they had been trained as such, and that they need not follow the norms of medical ethics.[126] Author I. Ahmad agreed: "A dentist providing cosmetic services should also accept that he or she is demoting himself or herself from the status of a professional to a skilled trader such as a hairdresser or tattooist."[127]

But for many dentists, cosmetic work felt like a natural extension of their practice. Practitioners had always been concerned with aesthetics – they prided themselves on the quality of their crowns and fillings and on matching tooth colours as closely as possible in partial bridges. Many whom I interviewed mentioned their work's artistic appeal as one reason they entered the profession.[128] Orthodontics had always been, at least in part, about dental aesthetics. As new materials became available, it only made sense to use them to enhance their work. As Dr Stephen Hancocks, editor in chief of the *British Dental Journal*, explained: "The replacement of the minimal amount of calcified tissue with a material which looks and functions as well as any non-natural material can, is the central activity of dentistry. It applies to everything we do."[129] The move towards cosmetic dentistry also fitted with the growing emphasis on customer service and patient empowerment. As Dr Ken Glick, a Toronto dentist and later president of the American Academy of Cosmetic Dentistry, observed in the JCDA:

> Today's average patient is more highly educated and aware of his or her wants and needs than ever before. Many come into my practice having thoroughly researched their options and being very knowledgeable about possible directions that their treatment might take. An ethical practitioner of cosmetic dentistry, like an ethical practitioner of restorative dentistry, listens to and understands the patient's concerns, takes a thorough history and performs a complete examination. When all of this has been completed, he or she provides a treatment plan based on the diagnosis derived from the information gathered. In most cases, he or she discusses alternative treatment modalities with the patient and compares the advantages and disadvantages of each. Then, and only then, having had professional guidance and advice, does the patient take responsibility for the ultimate treatment decision. The days of paternalistic medical or dental practice are past.[130]

Another defender, Alexander C.L. Holden of the University of Sydney School of Dentistry, commented: "The dental professional goals of yesteryear may have been firmly fixed upon alleviation of suffering. However, in the twenty-first century, it seems somehow denialist to suggest that the improvement of confidence and self-esteem is not part of the professional purpose of the dental profession."[131]

Conclusion

The desire for perfect white smiles dates back to at least the interwar years, when toothpaste ads featured smiling young women with "glistening teeth." The growth in orthodontics after the Second World War helped to create new expectations for what smiles could be. In the 1980s and 1990s, new techniques and materials made dentists even more exacting in their creation of perfect smiles. At the same time, many were reporting less-busy practices, and by the early 2000s new colleagues were graduating with huge debts.[132] This led many practitioners to adopt cosmetic work. At the same time, TV programs and magazines showed consumers what cosmetic procedures could accomplish. The demand for Hollywood smiles seems unlikely to diminish in the age of Instagram. In the process, dentistry has become less about health, or at least physical health, and more about beauty, confidence, and self-esteem. The pressures are greater on women, who have always faced more expectations around their appearance. Of course, the health aspects of dentistry have not disappeared, but the needle has shifted. This will change the conversation about dentistry's role in Canadian health care. If we embark on national denticare, what procedures should it cover? If orthodontics and tooth whitening are not included, what does this mean for people who cannot afford these treatments? As smiles become ever-more important at work and at play, how will this exacerbate inequalities in Canadian society?

Conclusion

Filling the Gaps

Over the past century, Canadians have seen remarkable improvements in their oral health. Today, three-quarters of them visit a dentist every year, and 84 per cent report good or excellent oral health. Their children have fewer cavities than the OECD average, and adults have lower rates of tooth loss.[1] These changes are due partly to a revolution in personal hygiene, made possible by rising incomes, better nutrition, affordable dental-hygiene products, and the spread of advertising, which promoted the use of toothbrushes and toothpaste. Advertising made bad breath increasingly shameful and white teeth a mark of success. Community water fluoridation in many cities helped slash tooth decay. Fluorides in toothpastes and oral preparations at the dentist's office reduced cavities even further. Increased access to dental treatment also makes a difference: the massive expansion in private coverage has led many people to seek regular preventive care, when once they might have sought assistance only in emergency.

But, as this book has made clear, substantial inequalities continue. People without private or public insurance find it difficult to obtain care, and even those with public coverage may not be able to locate a willing dentist, who will receive less than what private insurers will pay. People with disabilities are not always well-served by private dental offices, and many people living in long-term care lack oral health care.[2] Far too many children, especially Indigenous ones, suffer from dental decay. Toothaches cost up to 2.26 million school days per year, and a third of all day surgeries performed on young people aged 1–5 are the result of tooth decay.[3]

Currently momentum is growing for publicly funded dental care. In 2011, the Canadian Centre for Policy Alternatives produced a powerful report in favour of expanding access to dental care.[4] Provincial dental associations have undertaken a wide array of initiatives to improve oral health.[5] Over the past decade, British Columbia, Manitoba, Ontario, and Newfoundland all announced new investments in the area.[6] In Ontario, for example, "Healthy Smiles," started in 2010, provides free dental check-ups, cleanings, fillings, X-rays, and urgent oral health care for the roughly half-million children from low-income families.[7] The NDP included denticare in its 2019 and 2021 federal-election platforms. The Liberal government promised to improve access to dental care in its throne speech of January 2020. In October 2020, the Parliamentary Budget Office costed a program to provide dental care for all Canadians with a household income of under $90,000, similar to what Non-Insured Health Benefits provide Indigenous people.[8] Dentist Brandon Doucet and his Coalition for Dentalcare have lobbied hard for expansion of medicare.[9] The NDP made denticare a key demand in the summer 2021 election campaign.[10] But the federal budget of April 2021 included no new dental benefits.

The COVID-19 pandemic will probably complicate any expansion of dental benefits. Mounting deficits, the crisis in long-term care, preparing for future pandemics, and the move to green the economy leaves little room for new dental programs. Any advances are made harder by dentistry's strong cosmetic focus. Can we, or should we, separate physical health from medical interventions that make us feel better about ourselves? Many patients want straight teeth, white fillings, dental implants, veneers, and tooth whitening. For some severe dental problems, these procedures seem necessary. With others, they might help with employment and self-esteem. How does a public system distinguish between the essential and the purely "cosmetic"?

What is the best way to increase access to oral health care for everyone? One option is universal coverage, similar to what Canadians currently enjoy for hospital and physician care, with government the single payer. As with medicare, such a system is likely to gain broad-based support, while more targeted interventions, such as the post-1945 expansion of services to designated groups, are liable to cuts at times of fiscal retrenchment. From this perspective, a universal system has much to recommend it. But as this book makes clear, wealthier people seek out dental care more frequently than the less affluent, even if they all have access to insurance coverage. Thus universal coverage may well be regressive: those most able to pay for care are the ones most likely to seek it. A 2015 review of public spending on dental health across the country concluded that targeted interventions made the most sense, with some populations best served in the private dental office, and others, such as those in long-term care, receiving public care.[11]

In *The Politics of Dental Care in Canada* (2021), Carlos Quiñonez argues for a broad array of measures, including requiring all employers to provide dental benefits. He emphasizes that reducing social inequality by increasing income security, expanding educational opportunities, taxing sugar, and focusing on the social determinants of health will all improve oral health. He argues for specific interventions like fluoride varnish, dental sealants, and HPV vaccination (to prevent oral cancer). Universality, he points out, does not require a single payer like medicare but might mix public and private providers.[12] This option would be cheaper for governments, and potentially more appealing politically.

As this book shows, alternative providers can increase access to care. In the 1960s, when Canada was planning to expand health spending, most provinces decided to focus on children. This approach still has merit today, especially with cavities increasing after many decades of decline.[13] This change may reflect less water fluoridation, growing use of bottled water, as well as other nutritional shifts.[14] School dental clinics, like Saskatchewan's in the 1970s and 1980s, could well care for the largest number of children. Oral health professionals, like dental hygienists and therapists, could staff these clinics at less cost than dentists. Such facilities would help working parents, ensure care for all children, and ideally encourage lifelong pursuit of oral health.

Many adult Canadians cannot afford a dentist, while others cannot manage the travel or find the right practitioner. Long-term-care facilities still desperately need oral health care. Here, dental hygienists could play a vital role. Clinics for uninsured seniors who live at home could also improve oral health. We still need to expand access to rural areas, especially for people with disabilities or who do not drive. Mobile clinics, some of which already exist, could help significantly. We also must ensure opportunities for the working poor to obtain care. Even for people with public insurance, the current multiplicity of programs makes the system difficult for both dentists and patients. Simplifying the pathways to care could make a big difference.[15]

Attending dental school has become extremely expensive, and many graduates carry large debts. Setting up an office is not cheap, although many novices associate with a more experienced colleague for a few years. In a 2003–04 survey, very few students expressed interest in salaried public-health positions, and those who did were deterred by their debts.[16] As this book explains, many dentists revel in their role as businesspeople and feel lucky to have escaped the restrictions that face doctors who work under medicare. Over the past forty years, many dentists have focused increasingly on cosmetic, money-making procedures. Dental schools will need to pay more attention to health inequities and admit students from a wider variety of backgrounds, and government should provide incentives, such as debt forgiveness for recent graduates who are interested in careers in public health dentistry.

There is a great deal to celebrate about Canada's improved oral health. Many people keep their teeth for a lifetime. Fewer youngsters have mouths full of cavities, and far fewer people experience pain in their mouths. For some Canadians, going to the dentist has become a pleasant experience. Many greatly appreciate how these professionals can improve their oral health and the look of their mouths and teeth. Yet we should not forget the gaps in care. Too many people go without care, with damaging consequences for their oral health and their health overall. Too many go to the emergency department for urgent oral health care that a dentist could address more effectively and less expensively. To truly complete medicare, Canadians need to eradicate the smile gap.

Notes

Introduction

1 Nutrition Canada, *Dental Report* (Ottawa: National Health and Welfare, 1977) – research was done in the early 1970s.

2 Health Canada, *Canadian Oral Health Measures Survey* (Ottawa: Minister of Health, 2010), 33, 83.

3 H.K. Brown, H.R. McLaren, G.H. Josie, and B.J. Stewart, "The Brantford-Sarnia–Stratford Fluoridation Caries Study 1955 Report," *Canadian Journal of Public Health* 47, no. 4 (April 1956): 152.

4 Canadian Institute for Health Information, *Treatment of Preventable Dental Cavities in Preschoolers: A Focus on Day Surgery under General Anesthesia* (Ottawa: Canadian Institute for Health Information, 2015), vii, https://secure.cihi.ca/free_products/Dental_Caries_Report_en_web.pdf <4 Sept. 2021>.

5 Catherine Carstairs and Ian Mosby, "Colonial Extractions: Oral Health Care and Indigenous Peoples in Canada, 1945–1979," *Canadian Historical Review* 101, no. 2 (2020): 192–216; Ian Mosby and Catherine Carstairs, "Federal Policies Undermine Indigenous Dental Health," *Policy Options*, 5 October 2018, https://policyoptions.irpp.org/magazines/october-2018/federal-policies-undermine-indigenous-dental-health/ <4 Sept. 2021>.

6 Richard Barnett, *The Smile Stealers* (London: Thames and Hudson, 2017), 26.

7 Xiaojing Li, Kristin M. Kollveit, Leif Tronstad, and Ingar Olsen, "Systemic Diseases Caused by Oral Infection," *Clinical Microbiology Reviews* 13, no. 4 (2000): 547–58; "Oral Health–Systemic Health: What Is the True Connection?," *JCDA* 73, no, 3 (2007): 211–16.

8 Arlie Hochschild, *The Managed Heart: The Commercialization of Human Feeling* (Berkeley: University of California Press, 1983).

9 Loretta Kerr, "More Than Just Pulling Teeth: The Impact of Dental Care on Patients' Lived Experiences," *JCDA* 84 (2018): i4.

10 Peter Ward, *The Clean Body: A Modern History* (Montreal and Kingston: McGill-Queen's University Press, 2019); Katharine Ashenburg, *The Dirt on Clean: An Unsanitized History* (Toronto: Vintage Canada, 2010); Jean-Pierre Goubert, *The Conquest of Water: The Advent of Health in the Industrial Age* (Princeton, NJ: Princeton University Press, 1989).
11 M. Mendelsohn, *Canadians' Thoughts on Their Health Care System: Preserving the Canadian Model through Innovation* (Ottawa: Commission on the Future of Health Care in Canada, 2002).
12 Statistic Canada, "Canadian Health Measures Survey," https://www.canada.ca/en/health-canada/services/healthy-living/reports-publications/oral-health/canadian-health-measures-survey.html <13 May 2020>.
13 Donald Gullett, *A History of Dentistry in Canada* (Toronto: University of Toronto Press, 1971).
14 James W. Shosenberg, *The Rise of the Ontario Dental Association: 150 Years of Organized Dentistry* (Toronto: Ontario Dental Association, 2017); H.R. Maclean, *A History of Dentistry in Alberta, 1880–1980* (Edmonton: Alberta Dental Association, 1987).
15 Mervyn A. Rogers, *A History of the McGill Dental School* (Montreal: Faculty of Dentistry, 1980); Oskar Sykora, *Maritime Dental College and the Dalhousie Faculty of Dentistry: A History* (Halifax: Dalhousie University Faculty of Dentistry and the Nova Scotia Dental Association, 1991).
16 Carlos Quiñonez, *The Politics of Dental Care in Canada* (Toronto: Canadian Scholars, 2011); Souad Msefer-Laroussi, "Analyse du système de couverture de services dentaires au Quebec" (PhD diss., Université de Montréal, 2007).
17 Tracey L. Adams, *A Dentist and A Gentleman: Gender and the Rise of Dentistry in Ontario* (Toronto: University of Toronto Press, 2000).
18 Tracey L. Adams, "Interprofessional Conflict and Professionalization: Dentistry and Dental Hygiene in Ontario," *Social Science and Medicine* 58, no. 11 (2004): 2243–52; Tracey L. Adams, "Feminization of Professions: The Case of Women in Dentistry," *Canadian Journal of Sociology* 30, no. 1 (2005): 71–94; Tracey L. Adams, "'A Real Girl and a Real Dentist': Ontario Women Dental Graduates of the 1920s," *Historical Studies in Education* 16, no. 2 (2004): 315–38. Tracey L. Adams, *Regulating Professions: The Emergence of Professional Self Regulation in Four Canadian Provinces* (Toronto: University of Toronto Press, 2018).
19 Ruth Roy Harris, *Dental Science in a New Age: A History of the National Institute of Dental Research* (Rockville, MD: Montrose Press, 1989); Colin Jones, *The Smile Revolution in 18th Century France* (Oxford: Oxford University Press, 2014); Barnett, *The Smile Stealers*.
20 Sarah Nettleton, *Power, Pain and Dentistry* (Maidenhead, Berks.: Open University Press, 1985).

21 Alyssa Picard, *Making the American Mouth: Dentists and Public Health in the Twentieth Century* (New Brunswick, NJ: Rutgers University Press, 2009).

22 For an excellent account of this transition, by two of its instigators, see Susan M. Reverby and David Rosner, "'Beyond the Great Doctors,' Revisited: A Generation of the 'New' Social History of Medicine," in John Harley Warner and Frank Huisman, eds, *Locating Medical History: The Stories and Their Meanings* (Baltimore: John Hopkins University Press, 2004), 167–93.

23 Geoffrey Bilson, *A Darkened House: Cholera in Nineteenth-century Canada* (Toronto: University of Toronto Press, 1980); Paul David Gagan and Rosemary Ruth Gagan, *For Patients of Moderate Means: A Social History of the Voluntary Public General Hospital in Canada, 1890–1950* (Montreal: McGill-Queen's University Press, 2002); Wendy Mitchinson, *The Nature of Their Bodies: Women and Their Doctors in Victorian Canada* (Toronto: University of Toronto Press, 1994).

24 Maureen Lux, *Separate Beds: A History of Indian Hospitals in Canada, 1920s–1980s* (Toronto: University of Toronto Press, 2016); Esyllt Jones, *Influenza 1918: Disease, Death and Struggle in Winnipeg* (Toronto: University of Toronto Press, 2007); Erika Dyck, *Facing Eugenics: Reproduction, Sterilization and the Politics of Choice* (Toronto: University of Toronto Press, 2013).

25 Malcolm Taylor, *Health Insurance and Canadian Public Policy: The Seven Decisions That Created the Canadian Health Insurance System and Their Outcomes* (Montreal: McGill-Queen's University Press, 2009); David Naylor, *Private Practice, Public Payment: Canadian Medicine and the Politics of Health Insurance, 1911–1966* (Montreal: McGill-Queen's University Press, 1986); Gregory Marchildon, *Making Medicare: New Perspectives on the History of Medicare in Canada* (Toronto: Institute of Public Administration of Canada Series in Public Management, 2012); Delia Gavrus, James Hanley, and Esyllt Jones, *Medicare's Histories: Origins, Omissions and Opportunities* (Winnipeg: University of Manitoba Press, Forthcoming).

26 Gerard Boychuk, *National Health Insurance in the United States and Canada: Race, Territory and the Roots of Difference* (Washington, DC: Georgetown University Press, 2008); Antonia Maioni, *Parting at the Crossroads: The Emergence of Health Insurance in the United States and Canada* (Princeton, NJ: Princeton University Press, 1998).

27 Esyllt Jones, *Radical Medicine: The International Origins of Health Care in Canada* (Winnipeg: ARP Press, 2019).

28 Beatrix Hoffman, *Health Care for Some: Rights and Rationing in the United States since 1930* (Chicago: University of Chicago Press, 2012).

29 Sasha Mullally and David Wright, *Foreign Practices: Immigrant Doctors and the History of Canadian Medicare* (Montreal: McGill-Queen's University Press, 2020); R.D. Gidney and W.P.J. Millar, *Professional Gentlemen: The Professions*

in 19th Century Ontario (Toronto: University of Toronto Press, 1994); Jacalyn Duffin, *History of Medicine: A Scandalously Short Introduction*, 2nd ed. (Toronto: University of Toronto Press, 2010); Kathryn McPherson, *Bedside Matters: The Transformation of Canadian Nursing, 1900–1990* (Toronto: University of Toronto, 2003); Karen Flynn, *Moving beyond Borders: A History of Black Canadian and Caribbean Women in the Diaspora* (Toronto: University of Toronto Press, 2011); Pat Armstrong, Jacqueline Choiniere, and Elaine Day, eds, *Vital Signs: Nursing in Transition* (Toronto: Garamond Press, 1993); Myra Rutherdale, ed., *Caregiving on the Periphery: Historical Perspectives on Nursing and Midwifery in Canada* (Montreal and Kingston: McGill-Queen's University Press, 2010); Christina Bates, Dianne Dodd, and Nicole Rousseau, eds, *On All Frontiers: Four Centuries of Canadian Nursing* (Ottawa: Canadian Museum of Civilization, 2003); Jayne Elliot, Meryn Stuart, and Cynthia Toman, eds., *Place and Practice in Canadian Nursing History* (Vancouver: UBC Press, 2008); Cynthia Toman, *An Officer and a Lady: Canadian Military Nursing and the Second World War* (Vancouver: UBC Press, 2007); Susan Armstrong-Reid, *Lyle Creelman: The Frontiers of Global Nursing* (Toronto: University of Toronto Press, 2013); Peter Twohig, "'Are They Getting Out of Control?': The Renegotiation of Nursing Practice in the Maritimes, 1950–1970," *Acadiensis* 44 (2015), 91–111; Ivy Lynn Bourgeault, *Push! The Struggle for Midwifery in Ontario* (Montreal: McGill-Queen's University Press, 2006); Megan J. Davies, "Women Unafraid of Blood: Kootenay Community Midwives, 1970–1990," BC Studies 183 (2014), 11–36; Sasha Mullally, "Swedish Manual Training: The Macdonald Sloyd Fund and Education Reform in the Maritimes, 1903–1917," *Acadiensis* 49, no. 2 (autumn / automne 2020):159–71; Ruby Heap, "Training Women for a New 'Women's Profession': Physiotherapy Education at the University of Toronto, 1917–40," *History of Education Quarterly* 35, no. 2 (1995): 135–58.

30 Julien Prud'homme, *Professions à part entière : histoire des ergothérapeutes, orthophonistes, physiothérapeutes, psychologues et travailleuses sociales au Québec* (Montreal: Presses de l'Université de Montréal, 2011); *Histoire des orthophonistes et des audiologistes au Québec, 1940–2005* (Sainte-Foy: Presses de l'Université du Québec, 2005); Nadia Fahmy Eid, Aline Charles, Johanne Collin, Johanne Daigle, Pauline Fahmy, Ruby Heap, and Lucie Piché, *Femmes, santé et professions : histoire des diététistes et des physiothérapètes au Québec et en Ontario, 1930–1980* (Quebec: Fides, 1997).

31 Tracey L. Adams, *Regulating Professions: The Emergence of Professional Self-Regulation in Four Canadian Provinces* (Toronto: University of Toronto Press, 2018); Patricia O'Reilly, *Health Care Practitioners: An Ontario Case Study in Policy Making* (Toronto: University of Toronto Press, 2000).

32 Tracey L. Adams, "Education and the Question for Professional Status: The Case of Ontario's Dental Hygienists," in Elizabeth Smyth, Wyn Millar, and Ruby Heap, eds, *Learning to Practice: Professional Education in Historical and*

Contemporary Perspective (Ottawa: University of Ottawa Press, 2005), 265–90; Tracey L. Adams and Ivy Lynn Bourgeault, "Feminism and Women's Health Professions in Ontario," *Women and Health* 38, no. 4 (2004): 73–90; Tracey L Adams, "Professionalization, Gender and Female-dominated Professions: Dental Hygiene in Ontario," *CRSA / RCSA* 40 (2003), 267–89; Tracey Adams, "Attitudes towards Independent Dental Hygiene Practice in Ontario," *JCDA* 70 (2004), 535–8.

33 Catherine Carstairs, "More than Cleaning and Caring: The Profession of Dental Hygiene in Canada, 1951–2010," *Gender and History*, 22 Aug. 2021, https://doi.org/10.1111/1468-0424.12550 <29 Sept. 2021>.

34 Richard Wilkinson and Michael Marmot, *The Solid Facts*, 2nd ed. (Copenhagen: World Health Organization, 2003); Dennis Raphael, "Social Determinants of Health: Present Status, Unanswered Questions, and Future Directions," *International Journal of Health Services* 36, no. 4 (2006): 651–77; Paula Braverman, Susan Egeter, and David R. Williams, "The Social Determinants of Health: Coming of Age," *American Review of Public Health* 32 (2011), 387–8.

35 Alexandra Blair et al., "Identifying Gaps in COVID-19 Health Equity Data Reporting in Canada Using a Scorecard Approach," *Canadian Journal of Public Health* 112 (2021), 353–6; Adele Perry and Mary Jane Logan McCallum, *Structures of Indifference: An Indigenous Life and Death in a Canadian City* (Winnipeg: University of Manitoba Press, 2018).

36 Weston Price, *Nutrition and Physical Degeneration*, first pub. 1939 (La Mesa, California: Price Pottenger Nutrition Foundation, 2004). J.L. Bastos, R.K. Celeste, and Y.C. Paradies, "Racial Inequalities in Oral Health," *Journal of Dental Research* 97, no. 8 (2018): 881–2.

37 *Report of the Task Force on Misogyny, Sexism and Homophobia in Dalhousie University Faculty of Dentistry* (2015).

38 "Dentist Blazed Trails despite Racial Hurdles," *Vancouver Sun*, 8 May 1992, B3.

39 "'Gambling Gourmet Dentist': One of First Canadian-born Chinese Dentists Was Also a Top Table Tennis Player," *Province*, 17 May 2009, B3.

40 Evidence suggests that Jews entered dentistry in significant numbers because it had fewer racial barriers. In 1931, nearly 4 per cent of all dentists in Canada were Jewish, and the *Toronto Dental Yearbook* shows that many students belonged to the Jewish dental fraternity, Alpha Omega, through to the 1970s. Louis Rosenberg, *Canada's Jews: A Social and Economic Study of Jews in Canada in the 1930s* (Montreal: McGill-Queen's University Press, 1993), 194. Martin L. Friedland, *University of Toronto: A History* (Toronto: University of Toronto Press, 2002), 515.

41 My analysis of photos from the *Hy Yaka Yearbook* (1921–99) at the University of Toronto suggests that in the 1980s almost 20 per cent of graduates were Asian, and in the 1990s almost a third.

42 Brian Smedley, Adrienne Y. Stith, and Alan R. Nelson, *Unequal Treatment: Confronting Racial and Ethnic Disparities in Health Care* (Washington, DC: National Academies press, 2003).

43 Alison Mayes, "A Voice for Healing," *University of Manitoba Rady Faculty of Health Sciences Magazine* (winter 2018), https://news.radyfhs.umanitoba.ca/a-voice-for-healing/ <4 Sept. 2021>.

44 "Advertisement," *Oral Health* 70, no. 9 (Sept. 1980): 81; "Ski Whistler and Blackcomb: Tax Deductible Medical / Dental Seminars," *Oral Health* 79, no. 1 (1989): 70; "Seminar Marketing Services Inc. Announces a Few of Our Fall–Winter Courses," *Oral Health* 77, no. 10 (Oct. 1987): 62; "2003 Jasper Dental Congress," *JCDA* 68, no. 8 (Sept. 2002): 458.

Chapter One

1 W.R. Michell, "The Evolution of Health Service Work, Medical, Dental and Nursing in Schools in Toronto, with a Detailed Account of Its Growth and Present Status," *Public Health Journal* (Canada) 15, no. 12 (Dec. 1924): 541–56.

2 "School Children's Teeth in a Deplorable State," *Globe and Mail*, 30 Dec. 1910, 10.

3 W.H. Doherty, "The Dental Aspect of Medical Inspection of Schools," *Public Health Journal* (Canada) 3, no. 12 (Dec. 1912): 680.

4 J.C. Bayles, "False Teeth and False Hopes," reprinted from the *Independent*, *Maclean's*, 1 Nov. 1910, 96.

5 Shelley R. Saunders, Carol D. Vito, and M. Anne Katzenberg, "Dental Caries in Nineteenth Century Upper Canada," *American Journal of Physical Anthropology* 104 (1997): 71–87.

6 Jane Nicholas, *The Modern Girl: Feminine Modernities, the Body, and Commodities in the 1920s* (Toronto: University of Toronto Press, 2015), 6.

7 Mariana Valverde, *The Age of Light, Soap and Water: Moral Reform in English Canada, 1885–1925* (Toronto: McClelland and Stewart, 1991).

8 Nancy Tomes, *Gospel of Germs: Men, Women and the Microbe in American Life* (Cambridge, MA: Harvard University Press, 1999).

9 Booker T. Washington, *Up from Slavery* (New York: Doubleday, 1901), 174–5.

10 Sidney W. Mintz, *Sweetness and Power: The Place of Sugar in Modern History* (New York: Penguin Books, 1985); Richard Feltoe, *Redpath: The History of a Sugar House* (Toronto: Natural History, 1991).

11 Bettina Bradbury, *Working Families: Age, Gender, and Daily Survival in Industrializing Montreal* (Toronto: University of Toronto Press, 2007), 163–7.

12 Ibid., 91.

13 H.B. Anderson, "Diet in Its Relation to Disease," *Public Health Journal* 3, no. 12 (Dec. 1912), 708–13.

14 Caroline Durand, *Nourrir la machine humaine : nutrition et alimentation au Québec, 1860–1945* (Montreal: McGill-Queen's University Press, 2015), 31–55.

15 W. Peter Ward and Patricia C. Ward, "Infant Birth Weight and Nutrition in Industrializing Montreal," *American Historical Review* 89, no. 2 (April 1984): 324–45.

16 John Cranfield and Kris Inwood, "The Great Transformation: A Long-run Perspective on Physical Well-being in Canada," *Economics and Human Biology* 5 (2007): 204–28.

17 *Five Roses Cookbook* (Keewatin, ON: Lake of the Woods Milling Company, 1915), 5–7. For its popularity, see Elizabeth Driver, *Culinary Landmarks: A Bibliography of Canadian Cookbooks, 1825–1949* (Toronto: University of Toronto Press, 2008), xxvi.

18 Aubrey Sheiham, "The Epidemiology of Dental Caries and Periodontal Disease," *Journal of Clinical Periodontology* 6, no. 7 (1979): 7–14.

19 Clifford J. Baborka, "Diet in Health and Disease," *Journal of the Canadian Dental Association* (hereafter *JCDA*) 1, no. 2 (Feb. 1935): 67.

20 Ian Mosby, *Food Will Win the War: The Politics, Culture, and Science of Food on Canada's Home Front* (Vancouver: UBC Press, 2014).

21 Quebec. *Report of the Ministry of Health for the Years 1944, 1945 and 1946* (Quebec, 1948), 288–9.

22 Jean-Claude Moubarac et al., "Processed and Ultra-processed Food Products: Consumption Trends in Canada from 1938–2011," *Canadian Journal of Dietetic Practice and Research* 75, no. 1 (2014): 15–21.

23 Malvin E. Ring, *Dentistry: An Illustrated History* (New York: Harry N. Abrams, 1985), 166.

24 Allan Downey, *The Creator's Game* (Vancouver: UBC Press, 2018); D.W. Gullett, *A History of Dentistry in Canada* (Toronto: University of Toronto Press, 1970), 46–8.

25 Meryn A. Rogers, *A History of the McGill Dental School* (Montreal and Kingston: McGill-Queen's University Press, 1980).

26 Oksar Sykora, *Maritime Dental College and Dalhousie Faculty of Dentistry: A History* (Halifax: Dalhousie University Faculty of Dentistry, 1991).

27 Gullett, *A History of Dentistry*, 132–3.

28 Ian Sclanders, "Painless Parker: The Outlaw Dentist," *Maclean's*, 15 Dec. 1949, 7, 54–6; "A Brief History of America's Most Outrageous Dentist," *Smithsonian*, 28 Dec. 2016, https://www.smithsonianmag.com/travel/remember-when-pulling-teeth-was-fun-180960448/ <28 Aug. 2021>.

29 "News from the Provinces: British Columbia," *JCDA* 1, no. 2 (Feb. 1935): 87; "News from the Provinces: Manitoba," *JCDA* 1, no. 5 (May 1935): 230.

30 Ring, *Dentistry*, 308.

31 The first units were manufactured in the United States in 1913. By 1930, all dental schools offered courses in radiology. Few American dentists were using X-rays in 1925, but by 1930 46 per cent of new dental graduates purchased X-ray machines for their practice. See J.W. Stamm and R. Gilsig, *Recent Scientific and Technological Developments in Dentistry* (Montreal: McGill

University. 1976), 19–21; Vivien Hamilton, "X-Ray Protection in American Hospitals," in Brinda Sarathy, Vivien Hamilton, and Janet Farrell Brodie, eds, *Inevitably Toxic: Historical Perspectives on Contamination, Exposure and Expertise* (Pittsburgh: University of Pittsburgh Press, 2018), 23–49.

32 "Radiology: The First Hundred Years," *Oral Health* 85, no. 7 (July 1995): 20–1.

33 Malvin E. Ring, "W.D. Miller: The Pioneer Who Laid the Foundation for Modern Dental Research," *New York State Dental Journal* 68, no. 2 (Feb. 2002): 34–7.

34 "COPA Report," n.d. (c. 1932), Minutes of the Canadian Oral Prophylactic Association, University of Toronto Dentistry Library.

35 R. Dunlop, "A Condensed History of the Early Activities of the Canadian Oral Prophylactic Association," unpublished manuscript, University of Toronto Dentistry Library; Minutes of the Canadian Oral Prophylactic Association.

36 Wallace Secombe, "Editorial: A Relic of the Good Old Days," *Oral Health* 1, no. 10 (Oct. 1911): 256.

37 W.R. Greene, "President's Address to the Ontario Dental Society," *Dominion Dental Journal* 24, no. 7 (July 1912): 293.

38 Tracey Adams, *A Dentist and a Gentleman* (Toronto: University of Toronto Press, 2000), 94.

39 W.C. Gowan, "Tooth-Brushes, Their Proper Forms and Use, Instruction of Patients, Abuses of Mouth and Teeth Etc.," *Dominion Dental Journal* 18, no. 2 (Feb. 1906): 41–9; William J. Charter, "Ideal Tooth Brushing," *Journal of Dental Research* 4, no. 1 (March 1922): xi–xviii; Arthur H. Merritt, "Oral Prophylaxis in Its Relation to Preventive Dentistry," *Dental Cosmos* 61, no. 6 (June 1919): 473–9. The definitive work was Isador Hirschfeld, *The Toothbrush: Its Use and Abuse* (Brooklyn: Dental Items of Interest, 1939).

40 Alfred Fones, *Mouth Hygiene: A Textbook for Dental Hygienists* (Philadelphia and New York: Lea & Febiger, 1921), first pub. 1916. For its importance in the field, see Russell W. Bunting, *Oral Hygiene* (Philadelphia: Lea & Febinger, 1957), 6.

41 Provincial Board of Health, *Manual of Hygiene for Schools and Colleges* (Toronto: William Briggs, 1886), 177.

42 Severin Lachapelle, *Manual of Hygiene for the Use of School and Families Based on the Instructions of the Board of Health*, trans. M.T. Brennan (Montreal: Desaulniers & LeBlanc, 1891), 80.

43 *Leçons d'hygiène pratique à l'usage des familles et des écoles* (Montréal : Librairie Beauchemin, 1906), 94.

44 Cassidy Foxcraft, "Back to School … in 1915," *OISE Library News*, 8 Aug. 2017, at https://wordpress.oise.utoronto.ca/librarynews/2017/08/08/back-to-school-in-1915 <16 Oct. 2021>.

45 A.P. Knight, *Hygiene for Young People* (Toronto: Copp, Clark, 1911), 70–8.

46 Peter Ward, *The Clean Body* (Montreal and Kingston: McGill-Queen's University Press, 2019), 151.

47 The literature on focal infection includes Gilles Dussault and Aubrey Sheiham, "Medical Theories and Professional Development," *Social Science Medicine* 16 (1982): 1405–12; Jerry J. Herschfeld, "William Hunter and the Role of 'Oral Sepsis' in American Dentistry," *History of Dentistry* 33, no. 1 (1985): 35–45; Purnima S. Kumar, "From Focal Sepsis to Periodontal Medicine: A Century of Exploring the Role of the Oral Microbiome in Systemic Disease," *Journal of Physiology* 595, no. 2 (2017): 467; Paul Beeson, "Fashions in Pathogenetic Concepts during the Present Century: Autointoxication, Focal Infection, Psychosomatic Disease and Autoimmunity," *Perspectives in Biology and Medicine* 36, no. 1 (autumn 1992): 13–23.

48 Kumar, "From Focal Sepsis to Periodontal Medicine," 467; J.M. Vaizey and A.E. Clark-Kennedy, "Dental Sepsis in Relation to Anaemia, Dyspepsia and Rheumatism," *British Medical Journal* 25 (June 1939): 1269.

49 William Hunter, "Oral Sepsis as a Cause of Disease," *British Medical Journal* 28 (July 1900), 215–16.

50 William Hunter, "The Role of Sepsis and Antisepsis in Medicine," *Lancet*, 14 Jan. 1911, 79–86.

51 Beeson, "Fashions in Pathogenetic Concepts," 13–23.

52 Ibid., 13–23; E.C. Rosenow, "Studies on Elective Localization," *Journal of Dental Research* 1, no. 3 (Sept. 1919): 205–48.

53 Russell L. Cecil, *A Textbook of Medicine* (Philadelphia: W.B. Saunders, 1928), replaced Sir William Osler's *Principles and Practices of Medicine* as the authority in the field.

54 Ernest Hemingway, "Tooth Pulling No Cure All," *Toronto Star Weekly*, 10 April 1920, reprinted in Dateline Toronto; "Kiwanians Addressed by Dr. Winthrope," *Saskatoon Star Phoenix*, 6 Aug. 1920, 5.

55 Weston A. Price, *The Pathology of Dental Infections and Its Relation to General Diseases* (Toronto: Canadian Oral Prophylactic Association, 1916), 4–5.

56 Ibid., 14.

57 Weston A. Price, *Dental Infections, Oral and Systemic: Being a Contribution to the Pathology of Dental Infections, Focal Infections and the Degenerative Diseases* (Cleveland: Penton Publishing Company, 1923).

58 F.J. Conboy, "Dentistry as Public Health Activity," *Public Health Journal* 16, no. 6 (June 1925): 274.

59 H.W. Black, "Dental Hygiene," *Public Health Journal* 13, no. 9 (Sept. 1922): 416–19.

60 Ibid., 416–19. On Cotton's belief in focal infection, see Andrew Scull, *Madhouse: A Tragic Tale of Megalomania and Modern Medicine* (Cambridge: Cambridge University Press, 2005), 33–7.

61 William Osler and Thomas McCrae, *The Principles and Practice of Medicine* (New York and London: Appleton, 1923), 454.

62 Charles K.P. Henry, "Focal Infection," *Canadian Medical Association Journal* 10, no. 7 (July 1920): 598.

63 Ibid., 598–604.

64 "Meeting of the Halifax Branch of the Medical Society of Nova Scotia," *Canadian Medical Association Journal* 16, no. 4 (April 1926): 456.

65 "Tooth-Pulling Fad Not Cure for Ills, Dentist Declares," *Globe*, 27 May 1924, 11.

66 Hemingway, "Tooth Pulling No Cure All," 5.

67 "Early King's Aches, Famed Men's Deaths Blamed on Teeth," *Globe*, 14 June 1928, 14.

68 "Kiwanians Addressed by Dr. Winthrope," 5.

69 "Span of Life 58 Years Today," *Globe*, 6 April 1928, 13.

70 E. Thorburn Cleveland, "Dentistry – What Now?" *JCDA* 1, no. 7 (July 1935): 311.

71 Vaizey and Clark-Kennedy, "Dental Sepsis," 1272.

72 William J. Gies, *Dental Education in the United States and Canada* (New York: Carnegie Foundation, 1926), 36–7.

73 J.S. McEachern, "Greetings from the Medical Profession," *JCDA* 1, no, 1 (Jan. 1935), 13.

74 Canadian Dental Association Fonds (hereafter CDA Fonds), vol. 31, MG 28-1235, Library and Archives Canada (hereafter LAC); W. Cecil Trotter, "The Canadian Dental Hygiene Council Completes Ten Years of Successful Services," *JCDA* 2, no. 2 (Feb. 1936): 67–8.

75 Canadian Dental Hygiene Council, *Blazing a New Trail through the Rockies: Report of Mouth Health Campaign in the Province of British Columbia*, 1930, located in vol. 31, MG 28-1235, LAC.

76 "News from the Provinces: Manitoba," *JCDA* 1, no. 2 (Feb. 1935): 88.

77 "News from the Provinces: PEI," *JCDA* 1, no. 5 (May 1935): 232.

78 Sykora, *Maritime Dental College*, 222.

79 For example, in 1930, the CDHC distributed 40,000 copies of *Joy of Living* in Alberta as part of the campaign in that province. Canadian Dental Hygiene Council, *Annual Report of the Canadian Dental Hygiene Council*, vol. 31, MG 28-1235, LAC.

80 These were very similar to the instructions in the classic text: Alfred Fones, *Mouth Hygiene*, 2nd ed. (Philadelphia and New York: Lea and Febiger, 1921), 223–98.

81 Ontario Dental Association, *The Treasure House* (Toronto: Public Dental Health Committee of the Ontario Dental Association and the Canadian Dental Hygiene Council, c. 1925). For more on periodic health exams, see Catherine Carstairs, Bethany Philpott, and Sara Wilmshurst, *Be Wise! Be Healthy! Morality and Citizenship in Canadian Public Health Campaigns* (Vancouver: UBC Press, 2018), 117–21.

82 Ontario Dental Association, *The Joy of Living* (Toronto: Public Dental Health Committee of the Ontario Dental Association and the Canadian Dental Hygiene Council, c. 1925).

83 Canadian Dental Hygiene Council, *At the Gate* (n.d., c. 1930), vol. 31, MG 28-1235, LAC. In *At the Gate*, the text is identified as being based on R.M. Wilson, *How Our Bodies Are Made* (London, Henry Frowde, 1923).

84 The Department of Health, "The Health Guards," http://www.nanaimoladysmithretiredteachers.ca/index.php/skipsey-heritage-collection/mouth-health/ <28 Aug. 2021>. The department distributed 55,000 copies in 1930. Canadian Dental Hygiene Council, *Blazing a New Trail*.

85 Department of Health and Public Welfare, *Guard Your Health* (Winnipeg: Department of Health and Public Welfare, n.d.). Also available in WorldCat, published by Alberta Department of Public Health, n.d.

86 Dental Public Health Committee, Academy of Dentistry, *Champions Keep Fit: Do You?* vol. 31, MG 28-1235, LAC.

87 Bruce A. McFarlane, *Dental Manpower in Canada* (Ottawa: Queen's Printer, 1965), 83. Taken from M.M. Mehta, R.M. Grainger, and C.H.M. Williams, "Periodontal Disease among Adults," *JCDA* 21 (1955), 617.

88 Walt Disney, *Tommy Tucker's Tooth* (Laugh-O-Gram Films, 1922), https://www.youtube.com/watch?v=_5V2Wp-Isbw <28 Aug. 2021>.

89 *Bobby's Bad Molar* (1929), described in National Film Library, Catalogue of the National Film Library of Sixteen Millimeter Motion Pictures (Los Angeles: National Film Library, 1930), 43.

90 Donald T. Fraser and George D. Porter, *Ontario Public School Health Book* (Toronto: Copp Clark Company, 1925), 16–22.

91 F.J. Conboy, "Division of Dental Services," in *Annual Report of the Department of Health, Ontario 1925* (Toronto, 1926). 41.

92 F.J. Conboy, "Division of Dental Services," in *Annual Report of the Department of Health Ontario 1926* (Ontario, 1927), 35–8.

93 Ibid., 35.

94 F.J. Conboy, "Division of Dental Services," in *Annual Report of the Department of Health Ontario 1927* (Ontario, 1928), 51.

95 "Canadian Dental Hygiene Council: Report of Field Secretary," 6 Oct. 1943. in vol. 31, CDA Fonds.

96 F.J. Conboy, "Division of Dental Services," in *Annual Report of the Department of Health Ontario 1929* (Toronto, 1930), 56.

97 F.J. Conboy, "Division of Dental Services," in *Annual Report of the Department of Health Ontario 1930* (Toronto, 1931), 64.

98 W.G. Thompson, "Division of Dental Services," in *Annual Report of the Department of Health Ontario 1936* (Toronto, 1937), 93.

99 "Red Cross Gets Teeth Repaired," *Saskatoon Star Phoenix*, 6 Jan. 1923, 3.

100 Philip Dormer Stanhope Chesterfield, *Lord Chesterfield's advice to his son, on men and manners* (Vienna, 1799), 74.

101 William A. Alcott, *The Young Woman's Guide*, chap. 20, Project Gutenberg, https://www.gutenberg.org/ebooks/9054 <28 Aug. 2021>.
102 William Alcott, *A Young Man's Guide* (Boston: Perkins and Marvin, 1838), file:///C:/Users/ccarstai/Downloads/pg23860-images.epub <28 Aug. 2021>.
103 Wesley R. Andrews, *The American Code of Manners: a study of the usages, laws and observances* (New York: Andrews, 1880), 228.
104 *Bazar Book of Decorum* (New York: Harper and Brothers, 1870), 56–9.
105 Sophie Hadida, *Manners for Millions: A Correct Code of Pleasing Personal Habits for Everyday Men and Women* (Melrose, MA: Educational Service Bureau, 1932), 101–2.
106 Benjamin Gayelord Hauser, *Eat and Grow Beautiful* (New York: Tempo Books, 1936), 80–93.
107 Vincent Vinikas, *Soft Soap, Hard Sell: American Hygiene in an Age of Advertisement* (Ames: Iowa State University Press, 1992).
108 Kathy Peiss, *Hope in a Jar: The Making of America's Beauty Culture* (New York: Metropolitan Books, 1998), 97.
109 Kathleen Murray, "What Price Pulchritude?," *Maclean's*, 15 March 1932, 24.
110 Vinikas, *Soft Soap, Hard Sell*, 39.
111 Ibid., 129.
112 Letter from McGillvary Bros to COPA, 3 Nov. 1931, Minutes of the Meetings of the Canadian Oral Prophylactic Association, Dentistry Library, University of Toronto.
113 Barbara E. Mattick, *A Guide to Bone Toothbrushes of the 19th and Early 20th Century* (Bloomington, IN: Xlibris, 2010); Joseph H. Kauffman, "A Study of the Toothbrush," *Dental Cosmos* 66, no. 3 (March 1924): 300–13.
114 Stuart L. Fischman, "Oral Hygiene Products: How Far Have We Come in 6000 Years?," *Periodontology 2000* 15 (Nov. 1997): 7–14.
115 J.J. Mcarthy, "Bad Teeth vs. Good Health," reprinted from *Pearson's Magazine*, in *Maclean's*, 1 Oct. 1910, 119.
116 Joseph H. Kauffman, "A Study of the Toothbrush (II)," *Dental Cosmos* 71, no. 2 (Feb. 1929): 132–40.
117 Joseph H. Kauffman, "Original Communications: A Study of the Toothbrush," *Dental Cosmos* 74, no. 6 (June 1932): 601–6.
118 Elizabeth Hunt, *American Child Health Association, A Health Survey of 86 Cities* (New York: Child Health Association, 1925), xxiv.
119 Grant Dexter, "The Cost of Keeping Clean," *Maclean's*, 1 March 1933, 8.
120 Ontario, "Dental Conditions Found among Sample of 19,361 Ontario School Children," *Report of the Ontario Health Survey Committee* (Toronto, 1950), 187.
121 "Tamblyn," *Toronto Star*, 3 June 1936, 8; "IDA Drug Store," *Toronto Star*, 24 Feb. 1937, 15; "Pinder's," *Saskatoon Star Phoenix*, 2 May 1934, 7; "Liggett's," *Saskatoon Star Phoenix*, 14 Feb. 1935, 5.

122 "Tek Tells How to Avoid One Serious Misfit," *Maclean's*, 15 Dec. 1933, 32.

123 "Dr. West's Tooth Brush," *Globe*, 16 July 1923, 14; "Dr. West Tooth Brush," *Toronto Star*, 19 April 1928, 4; "Dr. West's Tooth Brush," *Toronto Star*, 12 Sept. 1924, 34.

124 "HI-GEN-IC Toothbrushes," *Globe*, 4 April 1924, 5; "HI-GEN-IC Tooth Brushes," *Toronto Star*, 28 April 1924, 25.

125 Pro-phy-lac-tic," *Globe*, 2 March 1923, 5; "Pro-phy-lac-tic," *Globe*, 9 March 1923, 14; "Pro-phy-lac-tic," *Toronto Star*, 8 April 1920, 9; "Pro-phy-lac-tic," *Saskatoon Star Phoenix*, 23 Aug. 1923, 10.

126 "Pro-phy-lac-tic," *Toronto Star*. 15 Oct. 1935, 43.

127 "All Leading Druggists Sell," *Globe*, 29 Oct. 1910, 12.

128 Dexter, "The Cost of Keeping Clean," 31.

129 With her "skin you love to touch" ads for Woodbury's soap in the 1910s, designer Helen Resor became one of the first people to introduce sex appeal into advertising. See Juliann Sivulka, *Soap, Sex, and Cigarettes: A Cultural History of American Advertising*, 2nd ed (Boston: Wadsworth, 2012), 104–8.

130 "Pepsodent," *Revue moderne*, Jan. 1925, 59.

131 Nicholas, *The Modern Girl*.

132 Pepsodent, "Pearls in the Mouth," *Canadian Home Journal*, Jan. 1922, 21.

133 Pepsodent, "They Have Found a Better Way to Clean Teeth," *Canadian Home Journal*, Feb. 1922, 47; Pepsodent, "Dents plus blanches en dix jours," *Revue moderne*, April 1924, 63.

134 Pepsodent, "During These Years, Mother, Take Them to the Dentist Often," *Chatelaine*, July 1930, 45; "Her Teeth Too Precious to Risk with Any Tooth Paste but the Softest," *Chatelaine*, April 1932, 33.

135 Pepsodent, "Irium Amazes Dental World," *Chatelaine*, April 1937, 3.

136 E.H. Hatton, L.S. Fosdick, and J. Calandra, "The Toxicity and Rubefacient Action of Sulphated Higher Alcohols," *Journal of Dental Research* 19, no. 1 (1940), 87–92.

137 Philip Kotler and Waldemar Proertsch, *Ingredient Branding: Making the Invisible Visible* (New York: Springer, 2010), 3.

138 Lyon's, "Do As Your Dentist Does – Use Powder," *Globe and Mail*, 22 Jan. 1938, 13; "Brighten Your Smile with Powder and Water," *Chatelaine*, Oct. 1942, 51; Bissell B. Palmer, *Paying through the Teeth* (New York: Vanguard Press, 1935), 146–50.

139 Pepsodent, "Davis Twins Confirm Laboratory Proof That Pepsodent Power Makes Teeth 32% Brighter," *Chatelaine*, Oct. 1942, 47. See also "Rick Twins Surprise Their Dentist," *Chatelaine*, July 1942, 26.

140 Palmer, *Paying through the Teeth*, 105. It is not clear if this campaign ran in Canada or not.

141 William Barrow, *Voice Over: The Making of Black Radio* (Philadelphia: Temple University Press, 1999), 35–46.

142 "Free … a 10-day Tube of Pepsodent," *Maclean's*, 1 March 1930, 33; "Germs Destroy Teeth and Tissues," *Chatelaine*, May 1930, 51. In her analysis of Aunt Jemima (the imaginary spokesperson for the Pearl Milling Company) advertising in Canada, Cheryl Thompson says that there is no record of Black Canadians protesting, although in Toronto Black protests in the 1950s did lead to the removal of racist books, including *Little Black Sambo*, from public schools. Cheryl Thompson, "'I'se in Town Honey': Reading Aunt Jemima Advertising in Canadian Print Media, 1919–1962," *Journal of Canadian Studies* 49, no. 1 (winter 2015): 205–37. For American protests against "Amos 'n' Andy," see Arnold Shankman, "Black Pride and Protest: The Amos 'N' Andy Crusade," *Journal of Popular Culture* 12, no. 2 (autumn 1978): 236–52.

143 Some of the images are available on this video put together by the Jim Crow museum at Ferris State University in Big Rapids, Michigan. https://www.youtube.com/watch?v=jVCI2WoZr1s <5 May 2017>.

144 Sherisse Pham, "Colgate Is Still Selling 'Black Person Toothpaste' in China," CNN *Business*, 19 June 2020, https://www.cnn.com/2020/06/19/business/colgate-darlie-toothpaste-intl-hnk/index.html <28 Aug. 2021>; Douglas McGill, "Colgate to Rename a Toothpaste," *New York Times*, 27 Jan. 1989, n.p.

145 "This Cleansing Foam Gives Teeth an Extra Protection," *Chatelaine*, April 1930, 37.

146 Colgate, "The Gleeful Smile That Greets You in the Morning," *Chatelaine*, July 1930, 39.

147 Colgate, "Why These Three Great Scientists Publicly Approve Colgate's," *Chatelaine*, April 1931, 31.

148 Palmer, *Paying through the Teeth*, 71.

149 Colgate, "The Gleeful Smile"; "Don't Live to Regret Half-Clean Teeth!" *Globe and Mail*, 12 Feb. 1930, 17; "Your Teeth Aren't Really Clean If You Only Polish the Surfaces," *Globe and Mail*, 12 March 1930, 16.

150 Roland Marchand, *Advertising the American Dream* (Berkeley: University of California Press, 1987). Sivulka claims that the Listerine ads started in 1922 and increased the firm's annual earnings from $115,000 in 1921 to over $8 million in 1928. See Sivulka, *Soap, Sex, and Cigarettes*, 184.

151 Colgate, "Fooled about Her Breath – and Never Knew It!" *Chatelaine*, Oct. 1935, 32; Marchand, *Advertising the American Dream*, 18–20.

152 Colgate, "Joan Gets a Job," *Chatelaine*. April 1937, 34; "Joan Gets a Job," *Saskatoon Star Phoenix*, 25 May 1937, 5.

153 Colgate, "If She's Coming Over – I'm Going Out," *Chatelaine*, July 1937, 35; Colgate, "Everybody Says He Neglects Me, but …" *Chatelaine*, Oct. 1937, 33.

154 "It Cleans Our Teeth and Makes Them Shine," *Chatelaine*, April 1938, 30; "Colgate's Is the Only Toothpaste Used by the Dionne Quints," *Chatelaine*, Jan. 1942, 24.

155 Colgate, "I Said 'No,'" *Chatelaine*, Oct. 1944, 30; Colgate, "Aw, Give a Guy a Chance," *Chatelaine*, Oct. 1945, 67.

156 Magda Fahrni, "The Romance of Reunion: Montreal War Veterans Return to Family Life, 1944–1949," *Journal of the Canadian Historical Review* 9, no. 1 (1998): 187–208.

157 Ipana, "Modern Foods, So Soft, So Rich, Threaten the Health of Your Teeth and Gums," *Chatelaine*, July 1929, 59; Ipana, "Never a Sound Tooth, Never a Healthy Mouth," *Globe and Mail*, 24 Oct. 1929, 17; Ipana, "Des gencives molles diminuent le charme de votre sourire," *Revue moderne*, Sept. 1941, 47.

158 Ipana, "'Appalling' Says Beauty Editor," *Chatelaine*, Oct. 1935, 3.

159 Ipana, "Another 'Dental Cripple' in the Making," *Chatelaine*, July 1937, 3; "Many Dental Troubles Are Due to Gum Neglect," *Globe and Mail*, 2 Oct. 1939, 8.

160 Ipana, "Q. Will he like my new coiffure?," *Chatelaine*, April 1941, 1; "It Takes a Pretty Smile to Sell a Song," *Chatelaine*, April 1942, 1.

161 Ipana, "Vous osez vous en prendre à mes gauffres," *Revue moderne*, Jan. 1946, 3; Ipana, "What! You Want Me to Stop Eating Stew?" *Chatelaine*, April 1945, 1; Ipana, "Say! You Act as Though Pastry Were Poison!" *Chatelaine*, April 1946, 1.

162 "For the Woman Who Makes Life More than Mere Routine," *Maclean's*, 15 June 1929, 76.

163 "Your Teeth Are Helpless," *Maclean's*, 15 Oct. 1932, 1.

164 "It's a Family Secret about Teeth," *Maclean's*, 15 Nov. 1932, 1.

165 Palmer, *Paying through the Teeth*, 245–51.

166 Lawrence B. Glickman, *Buying Power: A History of Consumer Activism in America* (Chicago: University of Chicago Press, 2009), 194–5.

167 Arthur Kallet and F.J. Shlink, *100,000,000 Guinea Pigs* (New York: Vanguard Press, 1933), 64–9, https://lithub.com/here-are-the-biggest-nonfiction-bestsellers-of-the-last-100-years/2/ <28 Aug. 2021>.

168 Stuart Chase and F.J. Schlink, *Your Money's Worth* (New York: Macmillan, 1936), 20.

169 McFarlane, *Dental Manpower in Canada*, 83.

170 Clifford J. Barborka, "Diet in Health and Disease," JCDA 1, no. 2 (Feb. 1935): 66–78; Mosby, *Food Will Win the War:*, 23–5; Harvey Levenstein, *Paradox of Plenty: A Social History of Eating in Modern America* (Berkeley: University of California Press, 2003).

171 May Mellanby and C. Lee Pattison, "The Action of Vitamin D in Preventing the Spread and Promoting the Arrest of Caries in Children," *British Medical Journal*, 15 Dec. 1938, 1079–82; May Mellanby, "The Influence of Diet on the Structure of Teeth," *Physiological Reviews*, 1 Oct. 1928, https://www.physiology.org/doi/pdf/10.1152/physrev.1928.8.4.545 <28 Aug. 2021>; Medical Research Council (UK), *Interim Report on an Investigation into the Influence of Diet on Caries in Children's Teeth* (London, 1931).

172 J. Menzies Campbell, "Is the 'Local Theory' Impermeable?," *JCDA* 2, no. 3 (March 1936): 105–10.

173 Russell W. Bunting, "Recent Developments in the Study of Dental Caries," *Science* 78, no. 2028 (1933): 420; "Russell Bunting," *New York Times*, 23 Nov. 1963, 29.

174 William A. Davis, "Dentistry and the Public Health Movement," in Walter J. Pelton and Jacob M. Wisan, eds, *Dentistry in Public Health* (Philadelphia: W.B. Saunders Company, 1949), 16.

175 William G.S. McLennan, "A Survey of Dental Practice," *JCDA* 3, no. 7 (July 1937): 364.

Chapter Two

1 "P&G: Crest Toothpaste 1950s," https://archive.org/details/dmbb36803 <30 Aug. 2021>. A longer version can be found on YouTube "Commercial – Crest Tooth Paste with Fluoristan – Look Mom, no cavities!," https://www.youtube.com/watch?v=VkDp3nC1Wyo https://archive.org/details/dmbb36803 <30 Aug. 2021>.

2 Peter Miskell, "Cavity Protection or Cosmetic Perfection? Innovation and Marketing of Toothpaste Brands in the United States and Western Europe," *Business History Review* 78, no. 1 (2004), 46–7.

3 Catherine Carstairs, "Cities without Cavities: Democracy, Risk and Public Health," *Journal of Canadian Studies* 44, no. 2 (spring 2010): 150.

4 Richard D. Lyons, "Decay in Teeth Will Disappear, Officials Predict," *Globe and Mail*, 26 Dec. 1983, 22.

5 Russell Bunting, "Recent Developments in the Study of Dental Caries," *Science* 78, no. 2028 (10 Nov. 1933): 419–24.

6 Margaret Cammack Smith, Edith M. Lantz, and H.V. Smith, "The Cause of Mottled Enamel," *Science* 74, no. 1914 (1931), 244. Of the first three studies, in Grand Rapids, Michigan, Newburgh, New York, and Brantford, Ontario, none initially used X-rays. Newburgh started using them in 1949, while Grand Rapids did some examinations with them beginning in 1946. Frank McClure, *Water Fluoridation: The Search and the Victory* (Bethesda, MD: US Department of Health, Education and Welfare, 1970), 119, 124.

7 H.V. Churchill, "Occurrence of Fluorides in Some Waters of the United States," *Industrial and Engineering Chemistry* 23, no. 9 (1931): 966–8. An excellent account of the McKays' efforts can be found in Donald McNeil, *The Fight for Fluoridation* (New York: Oxford, 1957).

8 H. Trendley Dean and Elias Elvolve, "Further Studies on the Minimum Threshold of Chronic Endemic Dental Fluorosis," *Public Health Reports* 52 (10 Sept. 1937): 1249–64.

9 H.V. Smith and Margaret Cammack Smith, "Bone Contact Removes Fluorine," *Water Works Engineering*, 19 Nov. 1937, in Howard Vernon Smith File, University of Arizona Archives. Thanks to archival staff for photocopying and sending me this material.
10 H. Trendley Dean, "Endemic Fluorosis and Its Relation to Dental Caries," *Public Health Reports* 53, no. 33 (19 Aug. 1938): 1443–52.
11 Kaj Roholm, *Fluorine Intoxication* (Copenhagen: N.Y.T. Nordisk Forlag, 1937), 138, 144; McClure, *Water Fluoridation*, 47–52.
12 D.A. Greenwood, "Fluoride Intoxication," *Physiological Reviews* 20, no. 4 (Oct. 1940): 582–616; F.J. McClure, "Nondental Physiological Effects of Trace Quantities of Fluorine," in Forest Ray Moulton, ed., *Dental Caries and Fluorine* (New York: American Association for the Advancement of Science, 1946), 88–9; Willard Machle, E.W. Scott, and E.J. Largent, "The Absorption and Excretion of Fluorides," *Journal of Industrial Hygiene and Toxicology* 24, no. 7 (1942): 199–204; Willard Machle and E.J. Largent, "The Absorption and Excretion of Fluoride," *Journal of Industrial Hygiene and Toxicology* 25, no. 3 (1943): 112–23; Frank A. Smith, Dwight E. Gardner, and Harold C. Hodge, "Investigations on the Metabolism of Fluoride," *Journal of Dental Research* 29, no. 5 (Oct. 1950): 596–600; Gerald J. Cox and Harold Hodge, "The Toxicity of Fluorides in Relation to Their Use in Dentistry," *Journal of the American Dental Association* (hereafter JADA) 40 (April 1950): 440–51.
13 H.E. Short, G.R. McRobert, and T.W. Barnard, "Endemic Fluorosis in the Madras Presidency," *Indian Journal of Medical Research* 25, no. 2 (1937): 553–68; H.E. Shortt, C.G. Pandit, and T.N.S. Raghavachari, "Dendemic Fluorosis in the Nellore District of South India," *Indian Medical Gazette* 72 (1937): 396–8.
14 Christopher Seller, "The Artificial Nature of Fluoridated Water: Between Nations, Knowledge, and Material Flows," *Osiris* 19 (2004): 182–200.
15 For example, Frank McClure, who did much of the early research on the systemic effects of fluoridation, discussed the Indian and South African studies in detail in "Nondental Physiological Effects of Trace Quantities of Fluorine," in Forest Ray Moulton, ed., *Dental Caries and Fluorine* (New York: American Association for the Advancement of Science, 1946), 84–5. This volume also contained articles on the situation in India and South Africa. McClure refers to the Indian studies in F.H. McClure, "Fluoride Domestic Water and Systemic Effects," *Public Health Reports* 59, no. 48 (1 Dec. 1944): 1953–8.
16 Paul C. Hodges et al., "Skeletal Sclerosis in Chronic Sodium Fluoride Poisoning," *Journal of the American Medical Association* 117, no. 23 (6 Dec. 1941): 1938.
17 McClure, "Nondental Physiological Effects," 90.
18 J.C. Burnham, "American Medicine's Golden Age: What Happened to It?" *Science* 215 (1982): 1474–9.

19 McNeil, *The Fight for Fluoridation*, 60; Ruth Roy Harris, *Dental Science in a New Age: A History of the National Institute of Dental Research* (Rockville, MD: Montrose Press, 1989), 109–10.
20 Roy Harris, *Dental Science in a New Age,* 78–9; David Bernard Ast, "The Caries–Fluorine Hypothesis and a Suggested Study to Test Its Application," *Public Health Reports* 58, no. 23 (4 June 1943): 858.
21 Clement Benson, "Open Wider, Please," *Maclean's*, 15 June 1943, 16.
22 Minutes, Health Insurance Committee, 6–7 Jan. 1950, box 14, MG 28, I235, LAC.
23 Alyssa Picard, *Making the American Mouth: Dentists and Public Health in the Twentieth Century* (New Brunswick, NJ: Rutgers University Press, 2009), 117–40.
24 A. Leroy Johnson, *Dentistry as I See It Today* (Boston and Toronto: Little, Brown and Company, 1955), 5.
25 Milton Nicholson, "The Practicing Dentist's Viewpoint," *JADA* 44 (Feb. 1952): 144–7.
26 "2500 Pediatricians Discuss Your Child's Health," *Chatelaine*, June 1952, 66.
27 F.A. Bull, "A Public Health Dentist's Viewpoint," *JADA* 44 (Feb. 1952): 147–8.
28 David B. Ast et al., "The Newburgh–Kingston Caries Fluorine Study," *American Journal of Public Health* 40, no. 6 (June 1950): 716–23.
29 "Fluoridation of Public Water Supply Now Urged by Research Scientists," *JADA* 41 (Aug. 1950): 211.
30 U.S. Congress, *Hearings before the House Select Committee to Investigate the Use of Chemicals in Foods and Cosmetics*, House of Representatives, 82nd Congress, 2nd Session, 1952, 1483–1803.
31 Juan M. Navia, "Dr. Robert S. Harris: Nutritionist, Oral Science Researcher and Visionary MIT Educator," *Journal of Dental Research* 77 (1998): 438–44.
32 Hearings, *Chemicals in Foods and Cosmetics*, 1524.
33 Ibid., 1491.
34 U.S. Congress, *Chemicals in Foods and Cosmetics*, 1602–14.
35 Letter from H.V. Smith to Robert Munch, 17 Sept. 1954, printed in Board of Health of the City of New York, Report to the Mayor on Fluoridation for New York City, October 24, 1955.
36 Statement of Dr Frederick Exner, Hearings before the Committee on Interstate and Foreign Commerce, House of Representatives, 83rd Congress, 2nd Session, on HR 2341, A Bill to Protect the Public Health from the Dangers of the Fluorination of Water. Fluoridation of Water (Washington, DC: Government Printing Office 1954), 62–86.
37 Waldbott is not mentioned in a hagiographical history of the American College of Allergists. Joseph A. Bellanti, "Proud of the Past: Planning for the Future," *Annals of Allergy* 70, no. 6 (June 1993): 445–61.
38 Nicholas C. Leone et al., "Medical Aspects of Excessive Fluoride in a Water

Supply," *Public Health Reports* 69, no. 10 (Oct. 1954): 925–36.

39 Rorty had published one of the first anti-fluoridation articles in the mainstream press: James Rorty, "Go Slow on Fluoridation," *Harper's Magazine* (Feb. 1953), 66–70.

40 F.B. Exner and G.L. Waldbott, *The American Fluoridation Experiment* (New York: Devin-Adair Publishing Company, 1957): 118–20.

41 *Fluoride* is published by the International Society for Fluoride Research, a coalition of anti-fluoridationists: http://www.fluorideresearch.org/ <20 April 2012>.

42 Robert L. Crain, Elihu Katz, and Donald B. Rosenthal, *The Politics of Community Conflict: The Fluoridation Decision* (Indianapolis: Bobbs-Merrill Company, 1969).

43 Dr K.A. Baird, "Fluoridate? First Weigh the Facts," *Canadian Doctor* (1969). Reprinted by the Canadian League of Rights, Flesherton, ON, pt 2, file 6769-3-1, acc. 1996–7/698, RG 29, LAC.

44 "New Help for Fluoridation," *Health* (summer 1974), page number obscured. The provinces subsidizing fluoridation included Nova Scotia (as of 1966), Quebec (as of 1967), New Brunswick (for much of the 1970s), Newfoundland (as of 1971), and Manitoba (in the late 1970s). "Water Fluoridation in Canada: A Status Report 1980," *Canadian Dental Association Journal* 47, no. 2 (1981): n.p.

45 "Fluoridation Plebiscite 'a Lot of Nonsense,'" *Winnipeg Tribune*, 28 Feb. 1962, n.p. (from Winnipeg Tribune Clipping Files, available on microfilm at the Millennium Library, Winnipeg); "A Tale of Two Cities," *JCDA* 21, no. 3 (1955): 179–80.

46 "Dental Conditions Affecting Children," A Report to the Canadian Conference on Children 1960 by the Canadian Dental Association, file 440-8-2, box 907, RG 29, LAC.

47 Doug Owram, *Born at the Right Time: A History of the Baby Boom Generation* (Toronto: University of Toronto Press, 1996); Cynthia Commacchio, "'The Rising Generation': Laying Claim to the Health of Adolescents in English Canada, 1920–1970," *Canadian Bulletin of Medical History* 19, no. 1 (2002): 139–78.

48 Letter from Joan McDonald to Ald. Mrs. Wilkinson and Gentlemen, 12 Feb. 1955, Council Minutes, 14 Feb. 1955, Calgary City Archives (hereafter CCA). This sentiment echoed in other places as well; see Letter to the Editor by K.D. Beardsall, *Globe and Mail*, 27 March 1959, 6.

49 See, for example, Brief #29, submitted by Roger Vallée, Royal Commission on Fluoridation, container 3, RG 18-140, Archives of Ontario (hereafter AO).

50 James G. Snell, *The Citizen's Wage: The State and the Elderly in Canada, 1900–1951* (Toronto: University of Toronto Press, 1996), 156–85.

51 Memo from Lloyd Bowen, Aug. 1978, Consumer Reports, pt 1, file 6769-3-3, box 87, acc. 1996–7, RG 29, LAC; John A. Yiamouyiannis, "A Definite Link between Fluoridation and Cancer Death Rate," pt 2, file 50-8-4, vol. 1784, RG 29, LAC. See also "Fluoridation: The Cancer Scare," *Consumer Reports*, July 1978, pt 3, file 6769-3-1m, acc. 1996–7/698, LAC.

52 Letter from Victor A. Cecilioni to J.J. Shekter, 18 April 1977, in pt 2, file 50-8-4, vol. 1784, RG 29, LAC; Richard Doll and Leo Kinlen, "Fluoridation of Water and Cancer Mortality in the U.S.A.," *Lancet* 8025 (1977), 1300–3; R.N. Hoover et al., "Fluoridated Drinking Water and the Occurrence of Cancer," *Journal of the National Cancer Institute* 57, no. 4 (1976): 757–68; *Fluoridation and Cancer: An Analysis of Canadian Drinking Water Fluoridation and Cancer Mortality Data* (Ottawa: National Health and Welfare, 1977).

53 "Why the Hurry?," *Globe and Mail*, 5 Feb. 1953, 6. Katherine Arnup shows that anti-vaccinationists also made arguments against compulsion both at the turn of the twentieth century and in the 1980s: Katherine Arnup, "'Victims of Vaccination': Opposition to Compulsory Immunization in Ontario, 1900–90," *CBMH / BCHM* 9 (1992), 159–76.

54 This is from a speech reprinted in Jean-Marc Brunet, *Dossier fluor* (Montreal: Éditions du Jour, 1972), 133–9.

55 Provincial Council of Women of British Council, "Fluoridation," pt 2, file 6769-3-1, acc. 1996–7/698, RG 29, LAC.

56 "Fluoride Pills," *Calgary Herald*, 8 Sept. 1966, 4; K. Pawson, Letter to the Editor, "Fluoridation," *Calgary Herald*, 13 Sept. 1966, 4; Leslie Morrison, Letter to the Editor, "Fluoridation," *Calgary Herald*, 21 Sept. 1966, 5.

57 Department of National Health and Welfare, *Fluoridation: One in a Million* (Ottawa, 1955).

58 Quebec, *Débats de l'Assemblé nationale* (19 June 1975), 1393 (Hon. Claude Forget, MNA).

59 Letter from E.S. Campbell to [Minister of National Health and Welfare] John Munro, MP, 24 Feb. 1971, pt 1, file 50-8-4, vol. 1783, RG 29, LAC.

60 Stanley Kubrick, dir., *Dr. Strangelove: Or How I Learned to Stop Worrying and Love the Bomb* (Hawk Films Ltd, 1964).

61 W.B. Herrstrom, "Twenty-five Reasons Why Community Water Supplies Should Not Be Fluoridated," *Americanism Bulletin* 17 (1951), 237, RG 128, LAC.

62 Sidney Katz, "The Bitter, Tragic Battle over Fluoridation," *Maclean's*, 16 April 1955, 20–1, 71–9.

63 Gretchen Reilly, "The Task Is a Political One," in John W. Ward and Christian Warren, eds., *Silent Victories: The History and Practice of Public Health in Twentieth-Century America* (New York and Oxford: Oxford University Press, 2007), 323–40; Gretchen Reilly, *"This Poisoning of Our Drinking Water": The American Fluoridation Controversy* (Washington, DC: George Washington University Press, 2001), 63–6.

64 See, for example, speech by Mrs. Lydia Arsens, MLA, BC Legislature, 22 Feb. 1955, circulated by the Pure Food Guild, file 21, series 101, 146-F-4, Vancouver City Archives (hereafter VCA). Brian Martin claims that ALCOA stopped producing fluorides in 1952. Brian Martin, *Scientific Knowledge in Controversy: The Social Dynamics of the Fluoridation Debate* (Albany: State University of New York Press, 1991), 213. The Aluminum Company at Arvida, which had once supplied Brantford's fluorides, stopped selling fluoride in the mid-1950s. D.B. Williams, "The Fluoridation of Drinking Water," *JCDA* 21, no. 12 (1955): 671.

65 Ralph Nader, *Unsafe at Any Speed: The Designed-in Dangers of the American Automobile* (New York: Grossman, 1965), helped galvanize a growing consumer movement in the 1960s. Nader also expressed opposition to water fluoridation.

66 Edwin Feeny, "The People Say," *Toronto Star*, 26 March 1961, 8.

67 N. Freeluau to His Worship the Mayor, 2 March 1957, in file 1, series 483, 35-E-4, VCA. Indeed, Vancouver had also had debates about chlorinating water. Matthew Evenden, "Debating Water Purity and Expertise: The Chlorination Controversy in Vancouver during the Second World War," *Journal of Historical Geography* 65 (July 2019): 85–95.

68 W.J. McCormick, "Fluoridation of Water," *Toronto Star*, 31 Dec. 1951, 6.

69 Iris Airth, "Water Fluoridation," *Globe and Mail*, 10 March 1961, 6.

70 Gertrude Fairburn to Marc Lalonde per J.R. Hickman, 13 Sept. 1976, pt 2, file 50-8-4, vol. 1783, RG 29, LAC.

71 Canadian Dental Association, "Nature's Way to Fight Tooth Decay," Nov. 1978, pt 2, file 6769-3-3, box 87, acc. 1996–7/698, LAC.

72 "Fluoride Count Indicates Town Water Safe: Dymond," *Winnipeg Tribune*, 30 Oct. 1967, n.p. (from Winnipeg Tribune Clipping Files, available on microfilm at the Millennium Library, Winnipeg); Letter to the Editor by K.A. Baird, *Daily Gleaner* (Vancouver), 30 Oct. 1967, n.p., file 6, series 483, 45-C-5, VCA.

73 Brief by Mrs Ruth Golman, an affiliated member of the Pure Food Guild of BC, n.d., pt 1, file 50-8-4, vol. 1783, RG 29, LAC.

74 Speech by M. Kwasnica, MLA, Cut Knife Constituency, March 1974, pt 3, file 6769-3-1, box 87, acc. 1996–7/698, LAC.

75 Carole Spindell Farkas, *Water Fluoridation: The Human Diet and the Environment* (Montreal: Society to Overcome Pollution, 1971).

76 Michael Egan, *Barry Commoner and the Science of Survival: The Remaking of American Environmentalism* (Boston: MIT Press, 2007), 47–78.

77 J.R. Marier et al., "Accumulation of Skeletal Fluoride," *Archives of Environmental Health: An International Journal* 6, no. 5 (1963): 664–71; J.R. Marier and Dyson Rose, *Environmental Fluoride* (Ottawa: National Research Council of Canada, 1977).

78 Jack Hann, "Environmental Fluoride 1977: A Critique," pt 1, file 6769-3-3, box 87, acc. 1996–7/698, RG 29, LAC; Canadian Public Health Association, *Criteria*

Document in Support of a Drinking Water Standard for Fluoride (Ottawa: Canadian Public Health Association, 1979); John Lear, "Documenting the Case against Fluoridation," *Saturday Review*, 4 Jan. 1964, 85–92; John Lear, "New Facts on Fluoridation," *Saturday Review*, 1 March 1969, 51–6.

79 Christopher Dummitt, *The Manly Modern: Masculinity in Postwar Canada* (Vancouver: UBC Press, 2008).

80 "Fluoridation – Yes!" *Ottawa Citizen*, 8 Dec. 1964, 17; Edmonton Election 2007, Election History, 1966, http://www.edmontonelection.ca/images/stories/pdf/results/1966.pdf <15 May 2008>.

81 Carstairs, "Cities without Cavities"; Public Health Agency of Canada, *The State of Community Water Fluoridation in Canada* (Ottawa, 2017), https://www.canada.ca/en/services/health/publications/healthy-living/community-water-fluoridation-across-canada-2017.html <30 Aug. 2021>.

82 Joseph C. Muhler, Arthur W. Radike, William H. Nebergall, and Harry G. Day, "The Effect of a Stannous Fluoride–Containing Dentifrice on Caries Reduction in Children," *Journal of Dental Research* 33, no. 5 (1954): 605–12.

83 Joseph C. Muhler, Arthur W. Radike, William H. Nebergall, and Harry G. Day, "Effect of a Stannous Fluoride–Containing Dentifrice on Caries Reduction in Children II. Caries Experience after One Year," *JADA* 50, no. 2 (1956): 163–6.

84 Joseph C. Muhler, Arthur W. Radike, William H. Nebergall, and Harry G. Day, "A Comparison between the Anticariogenic Effects of Dentifrices Containing Stannous Fluoride and Sodium Fluoride," *JADA* 51, no. 11 (1955): 556–9.

85 Miskell, "Cavity Protection or Cosmetic Perfection?," 29–60.

86 "Dentists Assail Some Ads on Toothpaste: Urge Congress to Force Proof of Claims," *New York Times*, 18 July 1958, 11.

87 "Crest," *AdAge Encyclopedia*, 15 Sept. 2003, https://adage.com/article/adage-encyclopedia/crest/98607 <30 Aug. 2021>.

88 Peter Bart, "Advertising: Ipana Adding Sodium Fluoride," *New York Times*, 28 June 1961, 25.

89 "Dental Association Gives Its Approval to Cue Toothpaste," *New York Times*, 31 July 1964, 28.

90 Philip H. Dougherty, "Advertising: Escalation of the Cavity War," *New York Times*, 1 Oct. 1968, 74.

91 Miskell, "Cavity Protection or Cosmetic Perfection?," 47.

92 Donica Belisle, "Anti-Black Racism in Food Advertising: Rogers' Golden Syrup and the Imagery of White Supremacy in the Canadian West," *Gastronomica* 21, no. 2 (2021): 14–27; Cheryl Thompson, "I's in Town, Honey': Reading Aunt Jemima in Canadian Print Media, 1919 to 1962," *Journal of Canadian Studies* 49, no. 1 (winter 2015): 205–37.

93 "Fewer Cavities. The Single Biggest Reason All These Families Use Crest," *Chatelaine*, July 1978, 96.

94 "This Child Could Grow Up Never Knowing a Cavity in Her Lifetime," *Chatelaine* 59, no. 5 (March 1986): 30.

95 "Why Do More People Use Crest's Tartar-Fighting Formula Than Any Other?" *Chatelaine* 60, no. 11 (Nov. 1987): 167.
96 Geoffrey Slack and Brian A. Burt, *Dental Public Health: An Introduction to Community Dentistry* (Bristol: John Wright and Sons, 1974), 28–30.
97 Geoffrey Slack and Brian A. Burt, *Dental Public Health: An Introduction to Community Dentistry*, rev. ed. (Bristol: John Wright and Sons, 1981), 32.
98 Brain A. Burt and Stephen A. Eklund, *Dentistry, Dental Practice, and the Community*, 6th ed. (Toronto: Elsevier Canada, 2005), 356.
99 Douglas Bratthlal, Gunnel Hänsel-Petersson, and Hans Sundberg, "Reasons for the Caries Decline: What Do the Experts Believe?," *European Journal of Oral Science* 104, no. 4 (1996): 416–22.
100 William H. Bowen, "Significance of Toothpaste in Oral Hygiene," in G. Emberty and R. Rolla, eds., *Clinical and Biological Aspects of Dentifrices* (Oxford: Oxford University Press, 1992), 9–12.
101 B. Krasse, "The Caries Decline: Is the Effect of Fluoride Toothpaste Overrated?," *European Journal of Oral Science* 104, no. 4 (1996): 426–9.
102 B.G. Bibby, "The Use of Fluorine in the Prevention of Dental Caries," *JADA* 31, no. 5 (1 March 1944): 317–22.
103 "Alternatives to Water Fluoridation," *JCDA* (Aug. 1961): 522.
104 Stanley Handelman and Domenick T. Zera, "Dr. Basil Bibby: Early Fluoride Investigator and Intellectual Provocateur," *Journal of Dental Research* 76, no. 10 (1997): 1621–4.
105 Burt and Eklund, *Dentistry, Dental Practice, and the Community*, 351.
106 Slack and Burt, *Dental Public Health* (1981), 25; Burt and Eklund, *Dentistry, Dental Practice, and the Community*, 351.
107 Flura-Tray advertised in *Oral Health*: "New from Kerr: Flura-Tray," *Oral Health* 62, no. 3 (March 1972): 43. At this time it came in orange flavour. "Premier Products" advertisement, *Oral Health* 67, no. 2 (Feb. 1977): 36. Today they're available in peppermint, grape, and cherry.
108 Robert Hawkins et al., "A Comparison of the Costs and Patient Acceptability of Professional Applied Topical Fluoride Foam and Varnish," *Journal of Public Health Dentistry* 64, no. 2 (2004): 106.
109 R. Gary Rozier, "Effectiveness of Methods Used by Dental Professionals for the Primary Prevention of Dental Caries," *Journal of Dental Education* 65 (2001): 1067; Amir Azarpazhooh, "Fluoride Varnish in the Prevention of Dental Caries in Children and Adolescents: A Systematic Review," *JCDA* 74, no. 1 (Feb. 2008): 73–9.
110 Hawkins et al., "A Comparison," 106.
111 "Fluoride Varnish: What Parents Need to Know," https://www.healthychildren.org/English/healthy-living/oral-health/Pages/Fluoride-Varnish-What-Parents-Need-to-Know.aspx <13 April 2020>.
112 "Alternatives to Water Fluoridation," *JCDA* (Aug. 1961): 523.

113 "Nutrition Committee, Canadian Paediatric Society, Fluoridation or Fluoride Supplements," *Canadian Medical Association Journal* 106 (22 Jan. 1972): 150–1.
114 Burt and Eklund, *Dentistry, Dental Practice, and the Community*, 347–8.
115 Per Torell and Yngve Ericsson, "Two-Year Clinical Tests with Different Methods of Local Caries-Preventive Fluorine Application in Swedish School-Children," *Acta Odontologica* 23, no. 3 (Jan. 1965): 455–60.
116 Dennis H. Leverett, "Effectiveness of Mouthrinsing with Fluoride Solutions Preventing Coronal and Root Caries," *Journal of Public Health Dentistry* 49, no. 5 (special issue, 1989): 310–16.
117 Stephen P. Kelin et al., "The Cost and Effectiveness of School-Based Preventive Dental Care," *American Journal of Public Health* 75, no. 4 (1 April 1985): 382–91.
118 Arnold Abramson, Terrance W. Hicks, and John Philion, "A Fluoride Rinse Program," *Canadian Journal of Public Health* 69, no. 2 (March–April 1978): 143–5.
119 James Morse Dunning, *Principles of Dental Public Health*, 4th ed. (Boston: Harvard University Press, 1986), 253.
120 *Annual Report of the Department of Health*, Ontario, 1980–81.
121 A. Ahaovuo-Saloranta, A. Hiiri, A. Norblad, M. Mäkelä, and H.V. Worthington, "Pit and Fissure Sealants for Preventing Dental Decay in the Permanent Teeth of Children and Adolescents," Cochrane Database of Systemic Reviews 2008.
122 Amid I. Ismail, "An Evaluation of the Saskatchewan Pit and Fissure Sealant Program: A Longitudinal Followup," *Journal of Public Health Dentistry* 49, no. 4 (Sept. 1989): 206–11.
123 D. Locker, A. Jokovic, and E.J. Kay, "Prevention. Part 8: The Use of Pit and Fissure Sealants in Preventing Caries in the Permanent Dentition of Children," *British Dental Journal* 195 (11 Oct. 2003): 375–8.
124 "The Dominion Dental Health Grants," *Toronto Star*, 26 May 1949, 6.
125 Ontario was the first in 1925, followed by Quebec in 1943, Manitoba in 1946, Saskatchewan, New Brunswick, and Nova Scotia in 1948, British Columbia in 1949, Prince Edward Island in 1950, Newfoundland in 1952, and Alberta in 1959. Quiñonez, *Political Economy of Dentistry in Canada*, 62.
126 La Ligue d'Hygiène Dentaire de la Province de Québec incorpore, ses réalisations, ses projets ; Campagne de propaganda et d'éducation en faveur de l'hygiène dentaire entreprise par la Commission d'hygiène dentaire du Collège des Chirurgiens-Dentistes de la Province de Québec, item 278, box 6, Canadian Dental Association Fonds, MG 28 I235, LAC.
127 C.A.E. McCabe, "To Instruct Lay Groups and Organizations in Dental Information," Minutes of the Committee on Public Relations, box 14, MG 28 I235, LAC. For more on Health Week, see Catherine Carstairs, Bethany

Philpott, and Sara Wilmshurst, *Be Wise! Be Healthy! Morality and Citizenship in Canadian Public Health Campaigns.* (Vancouver: UBC Press, 2018); H.K. Brown, *A Survey of Dental Public Health within the Dental Profession and within Public Health Agencies Including Those of Government* (Vancouver: University of British Columbia Faculty of Dentistry, 1969), 17.

128 Dental Public Health Committee of the Ontario Dental Association, *Your Baby's Teeth* (Ottawa: Child and Maternal Health Division, c. 1960), 4–5.

129 Ibid., 6, 18.

130 Vivian V. Drecnckhahn and C.R. Taylor, *Your Child's Teeth* (Chicago: American Dental Association, Bureau of Public Relations, 1940).

131 Dental Public Health Committee of the Ontario Dental Association, *Your Child and Mine: The Story of Dental Health* (Toronto, 1952).

132 The first edition was produced in 1951. Information Services Division for the Dental Health Division, *Dental Health Manual for the Use of Those Engaged in Teaching Dental Health* (Ottawa, 1958). The 1960 version was only lightly revised. Dental Health Division, *Dental Health Manual* (Ottawa, 1969).

133 The Ontario Society for Crippled Children was created by Easter Seals in the 1920s, http://www.easterseals.org/about-us/history <30 Aug. 2021>. One of the first uses of "dental cripple" is in Yes Fortier, Presentation to the Special Committee of the House of Commons on Social Security, 11 May 1943, in *The Dental Profession in Canada and Health Insurance: A Sequence of Presentations* (Toronto: CDA, 1944), in vol. 3, MG 28 I235, LAC.

134 National Film Board, *Something to Chew On* (Ottawa, 1948).

135 For mentions of fluoride in *Chatelaine*, see Elizabeth Chant Robertson, "Is Fluoridation Dangerous?," *Chatelaine*, Sept. 1954, 75. On teeth and beauty, see Eileen Morris, "Teeth Are Living Longer Too," *Chatelaine*, Feb. 1950, 47, 53; Elizabeth Chant Robertson, "Teeth and Teething," *Chatelaine*, Feb. 1952, 60. For *Revue Moderne*, see Alex Vallier, "Faites-vous une Âme printanière," *Revue moderne*, March 1960, 30; Claire Bertin, "Santé et beauté," *Revue moderne*, Oct. 1946, 17, 71.

136 F. McCombie, "Dental Public Health in Canada – 1960," *Public Health Dentistry* 21, nos. 1–2 (1961), 9–18. A description of the Victoria program appears in David Parfitt, "School Dental Inspection: Motivation Achieved by Four Different Methods of Referral," *JCDA*, (Jan. 1970): 32–4.

137 "La Ligue d'Hygiène Dentaire … "

138 Rapport annuel de la Ligue d'hygiène dentaire de la province de Québec inc pour la période du 1er avril 1965 au 31 mars 1966, vol. 6, MG 28 I, LAC.

139 Eunice H. Dyke, "Health Service in Schools," *Public Health Journal* (Canada) 13, no. 2 (Feb. 1922), 49–58.

140 Clarence Bouillon, "A School Dental Program," *Canadian Journal of Public Health* 42, no. 11 (Nov. 1951): 467–70.

141 McCombie, "Dental Public Health in Canada – 1960."

142 Canadian Dental Association, *Brief Submitted to the Royal Commission on Health Services by the Canadian Dental Association*, 1962, 19. See concurrence in *Brief Submitted to the Royal Commission on Health Services by the Royal College of Dental Surgeons of Ontario and the Ontario Dental Association*, 31, in vol. 3, MG 28 I235, LAC.

143 An account of the series as well as many of the clips can be found on Blogto. Ed Conroy, "That Time When the Toothbrush Family Came to Life," http://www.blogto.com/city/2013/03/that_time_when_the_toothbrush_family_came_to_life/ <2 May 2017>. On its CBC TV debut, see "CBC Buys Animated 'Toothbrush Family,'" *Canadian Dental Hygienist* 12, no. 1 (spring 1978): 5. The series (or perhaps a second series) aired on TV Ontario (TVO) through the 1990s; "TVO Short Programs," *Globe and Mail*, 26 Sept. 1998, D7. It also aired as part of the children's TV show *Captain Kangaroo* (CBS, 1955–84). "Aussie Created TV Toothbrush Family," *Toronto Star*, 26 Oct. 1977, E2.

144 Ontario Ministry of Health, *Murphy the Molar* (1972), https://www.youtube.com/watch?v=qLXAGztSPm4 <26 April 2017>; Ontario Ministry of Health, *Murphy the Molar* (1972), https://www.youtube.com/watch?v=dR4EElUrs7k <26 April 2017>. Both are available through the Archives of Ontario.

145 "Murphy the Molar Brushes up for Dental Health," *Toronto Star*, 20 April 1982, G16; John Keating, "Big Tooth Will Visit City Hall," *Toronto Star*, 9 April 1985, 2. A *Toronto Star* article on cuts to public health commented: "Murphy the Molar was as common in Ontario schools as Elmer the Safety Elephant and Smokey the Bear." Caroline Mallan, "Why Murphy the Molar Got Yanked," *Toronto Star*, 28 June 2003, F01.

146 Alan S. Gray and Diane Rothwell Hawk, "An Evaluation of a Grade One Dental Health Program," *Canadian Journal of Public Health* 59, no. 4 (April 1968): 166–8.

147 "Dental Health Week: Regina," file 6, box 1, R 913, Saskatchewan Archives, Regina.

148 "Self-interested Education in Prevention," *JCDA* 42, no. 2 (1976): 56.

149 Don Scranstead, "National Dental Health Month," *JCDA* 46, no. 3 (1980): 151.

150 Henry Meitkiewicz, "A Bigger Etobicoke Smile-a-thon Planned." *Toronto Star*, 15 Jan. 1976, B2.

151 William L. Hutton, Bradley W. Linscott, and Donald B. Williams, "The Brantford Fluorine Experiment: Interim Report after Five Years of Water Fluoridation," *Canadian Journal of Public Health* 42, no. 3 (March 1951): 81–7.

152 Michael E. Hamilton and W. Mark Coulby, "Oral Health Knowledge and Habits of Senior Elementary School Students," *Journal of Public Health Dentistry* 51, no. 4 (1991): 212–19.

153 Dennis H. Leverett, "Fluorides and the Changing Prevalence of Dental Caries," *Science* 217, no. 4554 (1982): 26–30.

154 Marian McDonaugh et al., "A Systemic Review of Public Water Fluoridation," NHS Centre for Reviews and Dissemination, University of York, 2000, https://www.york.ac.uk/media/crd/crdreport18.pdf <30 Aug. 2021>.

Chapter Three

1 "Dental Program Loss Still Painful in Towns," *Saskatoon Star Phoenix*, 12 May 1990, 4.

2 J.F. Conway, "Will Romanow Tame Business Lobby?," *Saskatoon Star Phoenix*, 22 Nov. 1991, 5; "Dentists Oppose Return to Former School Plan," *Saskatoon Star Phoenix*, 22 Nov. 1991, 12.

3 Michael Valpy, "Welfare: The Long (Wait) and the (Short) Benefits," *Globe and Mail*, 17 June 1970, 31.

4 Carlos Quiñonez and Paul Grootendorst, "Equity in Dental Care among Canadian Households," *International Journal for Equity in Health* 10, no. 14 (2011), 1–9.

5 Malcolm Taylor, *Health Insurance and Canadian Public Policy: The Seven Decisions That Created the Canadian Health Insurance System and Their Outcomes* (Montreal: McGill-Queen's University Press, 2000); David Naylor, *Private Practice, Public Payment: Canadian Medicine and the Politics of Health Insurance, 1911–1966* (Montreal: McGill-Queen's University Press, 1986); Gregory Marchildon, *Making Medicare: New Perspectives on the History of Medicare in Canada* (Toronto: Institute of Public Administration of Canada Series in Public Management, 2012); Gerard Boychuk, *National Health Insurance in the United States and Canada: Race, Territory and the Roots of Difference* (Washington, DC: Georgetown University Press, 2008).

6 Catherine Carstairs and Ian Mosby, "Colonial Extractions: Oral Health Care and Indigenous People in Canada, 1945–1979," *Canadian Historical Review* 101, no. 2 (June 2020): 192–216; Ian Mosby and Catherine Carstairs, "Federal Policies Undermine Indigenous Dental Health," *Policy Options*, 5 Oct. 2018, https://policyoptions.irpp.org/magazines/october-2018/federal-policies-undermine-indigenous-dental-health/ <1 Sept. 2021>.

7 Carlos Quiñonez, *The Politics of Dental Care in Canada* (Toronto: Canadian Scholars Press, 2021), 124.

8 Beatrix Hoffman, *Health Care for Some: Rights and Rationing in the United States since 1930* (Chicago: University of Chicago Press, 2012).

9 The Canadian public-health sector's spending on dentistry increased substantially in the late 1970s and early 1980s, reaching a high of 1.4 per cent of all spending in 1981, fell through the 1980s and 1990s, and has since stabilized at 0.5 per cent. National Health Expenditure Trends, 1975–2019, Series A, Canadian Institute for Health Information, https://www.cihi.ca/en/access-data-reports/results?query=dental&Search+Submit= <1 Sept. 2021>.

10 Carlos Quiñonez, "The Political Economy of Dentistry in Canada" (PhD diss., University of Toronto, 2009), 1–2; Canadian Centre for Policy Alternatives, *Putting Our Money Where Our Mouth Is: The Future of Dental Care in Canada* (Ottawa: Canadian Centre for Policy Alternatives, 2011).

11 Catherine Carstairs, "Medicare Unfinished: Pharmacare and Denticare," in Esyllt Jones, James Hanley, and Delia Gavrus, eds, *Medicare's Histories: Origins, Omissions, and Opportunities in Canada* (University of Manitoba Press, forthcoming); Catherine Carstairs, "Will Canada Finally Get Pharmacare?" *Conversation* (Canada), 31 Oct. 2019, https://theconversation.com/will-canada-finally-get-pharmacare-126248 <1 Sept. 2019>.

12 Naylor, *Private Practice, Public Payment*; James Struthers, *No Fault of Their Own: Unemployment and the Canadian Welfare State* (Toronto: University of Toronto Press, 1983).

13 John. S. Lapp, "Let's Think Nationally," *JCDA* 1, no. 5 (May 1935), 210–11. In 1935, at a meeting of the Eastern Ontario Dental Association, its president predicted: "State dentistry is bound to come in some form sooner or later." "State Dentistry Is Bound to Come," *Ottawa Citizen*, 10 Sept. 1935, 12.

14 "An Alternative to State Dentistry," *JCDA* 2, no. 4 (April 1936): 175–7; J. Gordon Coburn, "Looking Ahead," *JCDA* 2, no. 11 (Nov. 1936): 474; "The Coming Crisis in Dental Practice," *JCDA* 1, no. 2 (Feb. 1935): 83–5.

15 "Report of the American Dental Association Officials on the Practice of Dentistry under Compulsory Health Insurance Systems in Europe," *JCDA* 1, no. 12 (Dec. 1935): 555–6.

16 Ibid.

17 "Adequate Dental Care for the Masses," *JCDA* 5, no. 3 (March 1939): 179.

18 "Dental Statesmanship," *JCDA* 2, no. 12 (Dec. 1936): 557–9.

19 "Dental Institute of America," *JCDA* 2, no. 2 (Feb. 1935): 78–80.

20 Sylvister Moyer, "The Practice of Dentistry in the Drought Area of the West," *JCDA* 1, no. 3 (March 1935): 121–2.

21 Research Department, J.J. Gibbons Ltd, "An Analysis of, and Report upon a Survey conducted by the Toronto Academy of Dentistry," file 62, vol. 1, CDA Fonds, LAC.

22 "State Dentistry Move Supported," *Saskatoon Star Phoenix*, 31 May 1938, 10; "Dentists Propose State Dentistry," *Edmonton Journal*, 31 May 1938, 10.

23 "Think 90 P.C. in City Need Dental Work," *Calgary Herald*, 27 June 1938, 10.

24 Edmund A. Grant, "The Present Status of Public Dental Health Services in Canada," *JCDA* 5, no. 4 (April 1939): 214–22.

25 J. Gordon Coburn, "Looking Ahead," *JCDA* 2, no. 11 (Nov. 1936): 474.

26 H.K. Brown, "Where Are We Going with Dental Health Programs?," *Canadian Journal of Public Health* 48, no. 7 (July 1957): 281–4.

27 "Dentists Enter a New Age with Focus on Prevention," *Globe and Mail*, 30 Nov. 2017, https://www.theglobeandmail.com/partners/

advontariodentalassociation1117/dentists-enter-new-age-with-focus-on-prevention/article36860230/ <1 Sept. 2021>.

28 Don Gullett, *A History of Dentistry in Canada* (Toronto: University of Toronto Press, 1971), 192; "An Alternative to State Dentistry," JCDA (April 1936): 176; Canadian Dental Association, A Submission to the Royal Commission on Dominion–Provincial Relations Canada, 1938, 9–10.

29 Clement Benson, "Open Wider, Please," *Maclean's*, 15 June 1943, 16.

30 J.D. Adamson et al., "Medical Survey of Nutrition in Newfoundland," *Canadian Medical Association Journal* 52, no. 3 (March 1945): 227–50; Stewart MacGregor, "An Ounce of Prevention," *Health*, Jan.–Feb. 1948, 24.

31 S.L. Honey, "Our Dental Health Picture Is a Menace," *Health*, Sept.–Oct. 1948, 17.

32 Leonard Marsh, *Report on Social Security in Canada* (1943), reprint (Toronto: University of Toronto Press, 1975), 120.

33 Malcolm G. Taylor, *Health Insurance and Canadian Public Policy* (Montreal and Kingston: McGill-Queen's University Press, 2009), 47.

34 Principles for Dental Health Services Adopted by the Canadian Dental Association, in Canadian Dental Association, The Dental Profession in Canada and Health Insurance: A Sequence of Presentations, vol. 3, MG 28 I235, LAC.

35 Gregory P. Marchildon and Klaartje Schrijvers, "Physician Resistance and the Forging of Public Healthcare: A Comparative Analysis of the Doctors' Strikes in Canada and Belgium in the 1960s," *Medical History* 55 (2011): 203–22.

36 Presentation on the Subject of National Health Insurance for Dentistry in Canada, vol. 3, MG 28 I235, LAC.

37 "Says Rationing Helps Conditions of Teeth," *Globe and Mail*, 19 May 1943, 7.

38 "Warns against Regimentation," *Globe and Mail*, 31 May 1944, 7.

39 "Dental Service for Discharged Armed Forces Personnel," JCDA 11, no. 2 (Feb. 1945): 81–2.

40 Don Gullett, Report on the Dental Service under the National Health Service Act of Great Britain, vol. 14, MG 29 I235, LAC.

41 "Lower Incomes Bring Demands from British Dentists for Changes in Health Act," *Globe and Mail*, 8 July 1953, 8.

42 Charles Webster, *The Health Services since the War, Vol. I* (London: Her Majesty's Stationery Office, 1968), 363; Public Accounts Committee, 4th Report, 1950/1, paras 54–73.

43 Nairn Wilson and Stanley Gelbier, *The Changes in Dentistry since 1948* (London: British Dental Association, 2014).

44 "The Future of Dentistry in Canada," JCDA, 6, no. 10 (Sept. 1941): 451.

45 For a detailed description, see Taylor, *Health Insurance and Canadian Public Policy*, 1–68.

46 "The National Toothache," *Globe and Mail*, 31 Oct.1956, 6.

47 Statement of the Canadian Dental Association on the Recommendations of the Royal Commission on Health Services, 28 May 1965, *Transactions of the Canadian Dental Association* 1965, 35–8.

48 Ibid., 88.

49 "CDA Answers Royal Commission on Health Services," *JCDA* 31, no. 7 (July 1965): 462–3. It did recommend basic dental services for recipients of public assistance and their dependants. Statement of the Canadian Dental Association … 28 May 1965, 80–162.

50 For example, see John Harris, "An Ontario Perspective," in Conference Board of Canada, ed., *Dental Plans in Canada* (Ottawa: Conference Board of Canada, 1977), 29. Harris postulated that most people neglected their dental health, and that dental disease could largely be prevented if people acted appropriately, including voting for water fluoridation.

51 Canadian Dental Association, "Dental Health Plan for Children," *Transactions of the Canadian Dental Association* (1968): 215–89.

52 In Canada, 52 per cent of dentists employed an assistant. "Canadian Dental Association News," *JCDA* 10, no. 11 (Nov. 1944): 487.

53 James Leake, "Manpower Requirements and Cost Projections for Three Optional Models of Delivering Dental Care to the Children of Manitoba" (MSc thesis, University of Toronto, 1978), 19; H.C. Kilpatrick, "Production Increases Due to Chairside Assistance," *Journal of the American Dental Association* 82 (1971): 1367–72.

54 Tammy Thomson, "Shining the Light on Dental Assistants" (MA thesis, McGill University, 2015).

55 This was one of the recommendations by the Ontario Committee on the Healing Arts in its *Report of the Committee on the Healing Arts, Vol. 1* (Toronto: Queen's Printer, 1970), 20.

56 "Dental Hygiene Education, Licensure and Practice in Canada," *Canadian Journal of Dental Hygiene* 9, no. 3 (autumn 1975): 63.

57 Eunice May Edgington, "The Social, Economic and Political Influences on Women in Society and Dental Hygiene," thesis, University of Toronto, 1983, 7; D.W. Lewis, E.R. Wollis, and E.A. Lines, *Historical Trends in the Supply of Dentists and Dental Hygienists in Ontario, Research Report No.* 27 (Toronto: Department of Community Dentistry, June 1979), 13.

58 R.K. House, *Dentistry in Ontario* (Toronto: Queen's Printer, 1970), 86.

59 Leake, "Manpower Requirements and Cost Projections"; R.G. Romcke and D.W. Lewis, "Use of Expanded Function Dental Hygienists in the Prince Edward Island Manpower Study," *JCDA* 39 (1973), 247–62.

60 National Health and Welfare, *Ad Hoc Committee on Dental Auxiliaries Report* (Ottawa, 1970).

61 The Ontario Committee on the Healing Arts recommended that the Ontario Council of Health consider training and using dental nurses along the New Zealand and British models; *Report, Vol. 1*, 18.

62 J.T. Fulton, "Experiment in Dental Care: Results of New Zealand's Use of School Dental Nurses," *Bulletin of the World Health Organization* 4 (1951): 49–58; G.H. Leslie, *New Zealand School Dental Service 1921–1971* (Wellington: Department of Health New Zealand, 1971).

63 National Health and Welfare, *Ad Hoc Committee*, 13–20.

64 R.D. Holt and J.J. Murray, "Evaluation of the Role and Clinical Contribution of New Cross Dental Therapists," *Journal of the Royal Society of Medicine* 73 (March 1980): 187–8; National Health and Welfare, *Ad Hoc Committee*, 9–10.

65 National Health and Welfare, *Ad Hoc Committee*, 15–22.

66 H.H. Avent and H.K. Nikias, *Insured Dental Care Group Health Dental Insurance Inc.* (New York: Group Health Dental Insurance, 1967), as cited in ibid.

67 National Health and Welfare, *Ad Hoc Committee*, 24–5.

68 House, *Dentistry in Ontario*, 97; G.L. Woodward, J.L. Leake, and P.A. Main, "Oral Health and Family Characteristics of Children Attending Private or Public Dental Clinics," *Community Dentistry and Oral Epidemiology* 24 (1996): 253–9; J.L. Leake, P.A. Main, and G.L. Woodward, "Developing Evidence-Based Programme Guidelines for Children's Dental Care in a Dental Public Health Unit in Ontario, Canada," *Community Dental Health* 14 (1997), 11–17.

69 "Statistical Data – Dental Personnel," *JCDA* 20, no. 5 (May 1954): 281.

70 Malcolm Brown, *An Economic Evaluation of the Newfoundland and Saskatchewan Children's Dental Care Programs* (Calgary: University of Calgary, 1980), 3; Malcolm C. Brown, "The Public Finance of Medical and Dental Care in Newfoundland: Some Historical and Economic Considerations," *International Journal of Social Policy* 10, no. 2 (April 1981): 226.

71 *Canada Health Manpower Inventory* (Ottawa: Health and Welfare Canada, 1984), 42; *Canada Health Manpower Inventory* (Ottawa: Health and Welfare Canada, 1973), 32.

72 A.E. Chegwin, "Observation Mission to Study New Zealand Dental Program, July 1962," in *New Zealand School Dental Services: Reports of Observation from Saskatchewan* (Regina: Saskatchewan Department of Public Health, 1965).

73 Joseph J. Schachter, "The Dental Health of New Zealand Children, Adolescents and Young Adults," in *New Zealand School Dental Services.*

74 Paul Frederick Barker, "The Formulation and Implementation of the Saskatchewan Dental Plan" (PhD diss., University of Toronto, 1985), 48–69.

75 "Denticare Is Proposed by Saskatchewn CCF," *Globe and Mail*, 21 Nov. 1966, 17; Gregory P. Marchildon, "Access to Basic Dental Care and the Heavy Hand of History in Canada," in Canadian Centre for Policy Alternatives, *Putting Our Money Where Our Mouth Is: The Future of Dental Care in Canada* (Ottawa: Canadian Centre for Policy Alternatives, 2011), 20–3. In his dissertation (see n74 above), Barker argues that the College of Dental Surgeons of Saskatchewan had weak leadership in this era and that a questionnaire showed dentists actually fairly divided on the question of dental nurses.

Given the province's shortage of dentists, they also felt that they had little to lose. Barker, "Formation and Implementation," 108–9.

76 Preventative Dental Program and Recommendations prepared by the Dental Members of the Ad Hoc Committee and endorsed by the College of Dental Surgeons of Saskatchewan (1967). Found at Dalhousie Kellogg Library, Halifax.

77 *A Proposal for a Dental Program for Children in Saskatchewan*, Nov. 1972. Prepared by the Research and Planning Branch, Department of Public Health, Saskatchewan.

78 Steve Wolfson, "Use of Paraprofessionals: The Saskatchewan Dental Plan," in Eleanor D. Glor, ed., *Policy Innovation in the Saskatchewan Public Sector, 1971–82* (North York, ON: Captus Press, 1997), 129.

79 *A Proposal for a Dental Program*, 16, 20.

80 Ibid., 36.

81 Saskatchewan Advisory Committee on Dental Care for Children Report, 31 March 1973.

82 This was reprinted in other dental journals. Neil Munro, "Child Denticare – Saskatchewan," *International Journal of Orthodontics* 11, no, 4 (1973): 145–7; Neil Munro, "Child Denticare – Saskatchewan," *Journal dentaire de Québec* 11, no. 5 (1974): 4–5.

83 Research Committee of the College of Dental Surgeons of Saskatchewan, *A Dental Care Plan for the Children of Saskatchewan: Principles and Concepts* (N.p.: College of Dental Surgeons of Saskatchewan, 1973), ii–iii.

84 Ibid., 8–17.

85 Ibid., 16.

86 Ibid., 18–34.

87 Ibid., 39–45, 54–6.

88 Ibid., 53.

89 J.W. Stamm et al., *Dental Care Programs in Canada: Historical Development, Current Status and Future Directions* (Ottawa: National Health and Welfare Canada, 1986), 68.

90 Nick Hills, "Denticare Program Attracts Dentists," *Montreal Gazette*, 18 April 1974, 33; Stamm et al., *Dental Care Programs in Canada*, 67–72.

91 D.W. Lewis, *Performance of the Saskatchewan Health Dental Plan* (Toronto: University of Toronto, 1981), 65–6.

92 Stamm et al., *Dental Care Programs in Canada*, 68.

93 Garry Ewart, "The Saskatchewan Children's Dental Plan: Is It Time for Renewal?" (MA thesis, University of Regina, 2010), 81–2.

94 Ibid., 86.

95 Ibid., 90.

96 Ibid., 108–9.

97 Lawrence Thoner, "Changes Proposed to Dental Nurses Act," *Saskatoon Star Phoenix*, 6 May 1978, 21.
98 Ewart, "The Saskatchewan Children's Dental Plan," 113–19.
99 Gilles Dussault, "Dental Services in Quebec: Issues and Changes," *Social Science Medicine* 18, no. 3 (1984): 252.
100 Ibid., 252.
101 Ibid., 252.
102 Nova Scotia Children's Dental Plan, *Four Year Review, July 1974 to June 1978* (Halifax: Nova Scotia Health Services and Insurance Commission, 1980), Summary section, n.p.
103 Stamm et al., *Dental Care Programs in Canada*, 48.
104 Ibid., 69.
105 Lewis, *Performance of the Saskatchewan Health Dental Plan*, 73.
106 Brown, *An Economic Evaluation*, 19–21.
107 Ibid., 21.
108 Leake, "Manpower Requirements and Cost Projections," 76.
109 Susan Cartwright, "The Murder House Case Studies: An Education in Dental Anxiety" (MA thesis (Education), Auckland University of Technololgy, 2010).
110 Stamm et al., *Dental Care Programs in Canada*.
111 Peter Cooney, "Manitoba Dental Health Care Programs," *Canadian Journal of Community Dentistry* 3, no. 2 (1988): 38–40.
112 Stamm et al., *Dental Care Programs in Canada*, 56; Carlos Quiñonez, David Locker, Laurel Sherrett, Paul Grootendorse, Amir Azarpazhooh, and Rafael Figueiredo, *An Environmental Scan of Publicly Financed Dental Care in Canada* (Toronto: Community Dental Health Services Research Unit, 2005), 64.
113 Quiñonez et al., *An Environmental Scan*, 172–4.
114 R.G. Evans and M.F. Williamson, *Extending Canadian Health Insurance: Options for Pharmacare and Denticare* (Toronto: University of Toronto Press, 1978), 117.
115 Ibid., 122.
116 Ibid., 125.
117 D.W. Lewis, *A Comparison of the Experience of Children's Denticare in Four Canadian Provinces*, Prepared for the Dental Health Care Services and Epidemiology Research Unit, Faculty of Dentistry, University of Toronto, March 1977.
118 Shuance MacKinlay and David Rodenhiser, "Kids Dental Plan Cut Today," *Daily News* (Halifax), 1 Nov. 1996, 3, clipping file, Halifax Public Library.
119 Stamm et al., *Dental Care Programs in Canada*, 92.
120 James E. Leake, "The Ontario Dental Welfare Plan: A Success or Failure?" An Essay submitted to the Department of Dental Public Health in Partial Fulfillment of the Requirements for the Diploma in Dental Public Health,

University of Toronto, 1969, 6; "Canadian Dental Association Assails Fluoridation Critics," *Globe and Mail*, 21 March 1962, 13.

121 Stamm et al., *Dental Care Programs in Canada*, 81.

122 Ibid.; Leah Hamilton and James P. Mulvale, "'Human Again': The (Unrealized) Promise of Basic Income in Ontario," *Journal of Poverty* 23, no. 7 (2019): 576–99.

123 Stamm et al., *Dental Care Programs in Canada*, 81.

124 Leake, "The Ontario Dental Welfare Plan," 18.

125 Ibid., 29–33.

126 House, *Dentistry in Ontario*, 99.

127 "BC Dentists Withdraw Welfare Service," *JCDA* 34, no. 8 (1968): 456.

128 "Communiqué de l'APCDQ, La loi de la jungle – les assistés sociaux et les chirurgiens dentistes – Medicare imminent – Sommes nous prêts? L'impératif de la solidarité professionelle," *Journal dentaire du Québec* (April 1969), 14.

129 Stamm et al., *Dental Care Programs in Canada*, 60–4.

130 Claude Chicoine, "Dental Plans and the Dental Profession: A Quebec Perspective," Conference Board of Canada, *Dental Plans in Canada: A Growing Benefit* (Ottawa: Conference Board of Canada, 1977), 23–4.

131 Christophe Bedos, Jean-Marc Brodeur, Laurence Boucheron, Lucie Richard, Mike Benigeri, Marie Oliver, and Slim Haddad, "The Dental Care Pathway of Welfare Recipients in Quebec," *Social Science Medicine* 57 (2003): 2089–99.

132 House, *Dentistry in* Ontario, 91.

133 C. Bedos, A. Levine, and J.M. Brodeur, "How People on Social Assistance Perceive, Experience and Improve Oral Health," *Journal of Dental Research* 88, no. 7 (2009): 653–67.

134 V.E. Muirhead, A. Levine, B. Nicolau, A. Landry, and C. Bedos, "Life Course Experiences and Lay Diagnosis Explain Low-income Parents' Child Dental Decisions: A Qualitative Study," *Community Dentistry and Oral Epidemiology* 41 (2013): 13–21.

135 Christophe Bedos, Jean-Marc Brodeur, Alissa Levine, Lucie Richard, Laurence Boucheron, and Witnisse Mereus, "Perception of Dental Illness among Persons Receiving Public Assistance in Montreal," *American Journal of Public Health* 90, no. 8 (2005): 1340–4.

136 Christophe Bedos, Christine Loignon, Anne Landry, Paul J. Allison, and Lucie Richard, "How Health Professionals Perceive and Experience Treating People on Social Assistance: A Qualitative Study among Dentists in Montreal, Canada," *BMC Health Services Research* 13 (2013): 464–75.

137 Carlos R. Quiñonez, Rafael Figueiredo, and David Locker, "Canadian Dentists' Opinions on Publicly Financed Dental Care," *Journal of Public Health Dentistry* 69, no. 2 (2009): 64–73.

138 Carlos Quiñonez, Rafael Figueiredo, Amir Azarpazhoo, and David Locker, "Public Preferences for Seeking Publicly Financed Dental Care and

Professional Preferences for Structuring It," *Community Dentistry and Oral Epidemiology* 38, no. 2 (2010): 152–8.

139 Carlos Quiñonez, Luciano Ieraci, and Astrid Guttman, "Potentially Preventable Hospital Use for Dental Conditions: Implications for Expanding Dental Coverage for Low Income Populations," *Journal of Health Care for the Poor and Underserved* 22, no. 3 (Aug. 2011): 1048–58.

140 Margaret Neave, W. Harcus Inkster, and H.J. Philips, "Dental Care in an Institution for the Mentally Retarded," JCDA 37, no, 10 (Oct. 1971): 384–6.

141 Joan M. Rush, *Help! Teeth Hurt: Governments Obligation to Provide Timely Access to Dental Treatment to BC Adults Who Have Developmental Disabilities* (self-published), 66, https://www.bernardllp.ca/wp-content/uploads/2011/10/HelpTeethHurt.pdf <1 Sept. 2021>.

142 Anjani Koneru, "Access to Dental Care for Persons with Disabilities in Ontario: A Focus on Persons with Developmental Disabilities," MSc thesis, University of Toronto, 2008.

143 Carstairs and Mosby, "Colonial Extractions," 201.

144 S. Kamen, "History of Dentistry for the Handicapped: Past, Present and Future," JCDA (July 1971): 348.

145 "Access to Care: Ontario Universities Taking Action," CDA *Essentials* 2, no. 1 (2015): 35.

146 Norman Levine and J.A. Hargreaves, "Education as a Means to Prevent Dental Problems for the Handicapped," JCDA 43, no. 4 (April 1977): 185.

147 Joan Rush, "Treating Adults with Developmental Disabilities: A Mother's Call to Action," CDA *Essentials* 2, no. 1 (2015): 26–8, https://www.cda-adc.ca/en/services/essentials/2015/issue1/files/assets/common/downloads/publication.pdf <1 Sept. 2021>.

148 Clive Freeman, "Treating Adults with Developmental Disabilities: The Chairside Perspective," CDA *Essentials* 2, no. 1 (2015): 31.

149 A. Richardson and R.D. Atkins, "Normalization of Dental Care for Handicapped Patients in a Medium-Sized Canadian City: A Team Approach," JCDA 48, no. 6 (June 1982): 399.

150 Farnaz Rashid-Kandvani, Belind Nicolau, and Christophe Bedos, "Access to Dental Services for People Using a Wheelchair," *American Journal of Public Health* 105, no. 11 (Nov. 2015): 2312–17.

151 Rush, *Help! Teeth Hurt*, 10.

152 Ray E. McDermott and Hossam E. Elbdrawy, "A Survey of Parents' Perception of the Dental Needs of Their Handicapped Child," JCDA 52, no. 5 (May 1986): 425–7. Most dental offices in Ontario today are accessible for wheelchairs. Koneru, *Access to Dental Care*, 58.

153 "Handicapped Must Become a Priority and Not an Afterthought for Canadian Dentists," JCDA 47, no. 11 (Sept. 1981): 554–5.

154 Ibid.

155 Rush, *Help! Teeth Hurt*, 66.

156 McDermott and Elbdrawy, "A Survey of Parents' Perception," 425–7.
157 B.A. Richardson and R.D. Atkins, "Normalization of Dental Care for Handicapped Patients," 395; Norman Levine and Michael J. Sigal, "Dental Care for the Handicapped," *Canadian Family Physician* 35 (Feb. 1989): 370.
158 Koneru, *Access to Dental Care*, 29–30.
159 D.J. Kenny and J.S. McKim, "Dental Care Demand for Mongoloid and Cerebral Palsied Children," *JCDA* 37, no. 5 (July 1971): 270–4.
160 Anjani Koneru and Michael J. Sigal, "Access to Dental Care for Persons with Developmental Disabilities in Ontario," *JCDA* 75, no. 2 (March 2009): 121a–121g.
161 Warren P. Loeppky and Michael J. Sigal, "Patients with Special Health Care Needs in General and Pediatric Dental Practices in Ontario," *JCDA* 72, no. 10 (Dec. 2006–Jan. 2007): 915–915d.
162 Paul J. Allison and Herenia P. Lawrence, "A Paired Comparison of Dental Care in Canadians with Down Syndrome and Their Siblings without Down Syndrome," *Community Dentistry and Oral Epidemiology* 32 (2004): 99–106.
163 Koneru, *Access to Dental Care*, 73.
164 Clive Freeman, "Treating Adults with Developmental Disabilities: The Chairside Perspective," *CDA Essentials* 2, no. 1 (2015): 32.
165 Amin Salmasi, Rosamund Harrison, and Mario A. Brondani, "They Stole Her Teeth! An Exploration of Adults with Developmental Disability Experiences with Dental Care," *Special Care Dentist* 35, no. 5 (2015): 221–8.
166 Rashid-Kandvani, Nicolau, and Bedos, "Access to Dental Services," 2312–17.
167 Quiñonez et al., *An Environmental Scan*, 34.
168 Donald W. Lewis and G.W. Thompson, "Utilization in Alberta's Universal Dental Plan for the Elderly, 1974–1991," *Journal of Public Health Dentistry* 52, no. 5 (1992): 260.
169 Stamm et al., *Dental Care Programs in Canada*, 24–9; D.W. Lewis and G.W. Thompson, "Alberta's Universal Dental Plan for the Elderly: Differences in Use over Six Years by Two Cohorts," *American Journal of Public Health* 85, no. 10 (1995): 1408.
170 Lewis and Thompson, "Alberta's Universal Dental Plan for the Elderly," 1408–11.
171 Donna M. Wilson and Janet Ross Kerr, "Alberta's Deficit-Elimination Agenda: How Have Seniors Fared?," *Canadian Journal on Aging* 17, no. 2 (summer 1998): 206.
172 "Alberta Budget Cuts Kick in with Senior's Health Cuts and Premium Hikes," *Canadian News Wire*, 2 April 2002.
173 "Seniors' Income from 1976 to 2014: Four Decades, Two Stories," https://www150.statcan.gc.ca/n1/pub/11-630-x/11-630-x2016008-eng.htm <1 Sept. 2021>.
174 Barbara Yaffe, "Drill, Fill and Bill," *Globe and Mail*, 16 July 1979, 4.

175 "For Those Who Can't Grin and Bear It," *Globe and Mail*, 7 Aug. 1978, 6.
176 Nino Wischnewski, "Dentists Wouldn't Trade Their Freedom for MDs' Restrictions," *Calgary Herald*, 21 Sept. 1979, B4.
177 The number of Canadian applicants doubled from 1966 to 1971. Council on Education, Canadian Dental Association, *Applicants and Applications to Canadian Dental Schools* (Toronto, 1971), 4.
178 Yaffe, "Drill, Fill and Bill," 4.
179 Interview with D.B., 9 Sept. 2013; interview with L.T., 13 Aug. 2013.

Chapter Four

1 Mike Zettel, "Builders of the Community," *Niagara This Week*, 6 June 2011, 1.
2 David Naylor, *Private Practice, Public Payment: Canadian Medicine and the Politics of Health Insurance, 1911–1966* (Montreal: McGill-Queen's University Press, 1968), 135–75.
3 "Dental Post-Payment Plans," *JCDA* 18, no. 12 (Dec. 1952): 705–7.
4 "Saskatchewan Dental Services: Post Payment Plan," *JCDA* 27, no. 2 (Feb. 1956): 90.
5 "Group Purchase Plans for Prepaid Dental Care," *JCDA* 26, no. 12 (Dec. 1960): 722–3.
6 John Stamm et al., *Dental Care Programs in Canada: Historical Development, Current Status and Future Directions* (Ottawa: National Health and Welfare Canada, 1986), 95.
7 Ashin Khemani, *Canadian Group Insurance Benefits: A Practitioners Guide and Reference Manual* (Canadian Group Insurance Benefits, 2004), 7-1.
8 "Alberta Prepaid Dental Plan Described," *JCDA* 34, no. 7 (July 1968): 394.
9 "Alberta Corporation Offers New Prepaid Dental Plan," *JCDA* 35, no. 6 (June 1969): 292.
10 The CDA first warned about commercial insurance companies in 1964. *Transactions of the Canadian Dental Association*, 24–27 June 1964, 16; M.J. Lipkind, "Dental Service Corporation – Now!," *JCDA* 35, no. 5 (May 1970): 172.
11 *Transactions of the Canadian Dental Association*, 24–26 June 1968, 27.
12 Ibid., 7–9 July 1969, 26.
13 "Dentists, Lack of Plans Blamed for Disease, Neglect," *Globe and Mail*, 20 May 1969, 12.
14 *Report on the Findings of the Oral Health Component of the Canadian Health Measures Survey* 2007–9 (Ottawa, 2010), 12; James L. Leake, "Managing Dental Care versus Managed Dental Care: Looking South from North of the 49th Parallel," *JCDA* 64, no. 11 (Dec. 1998): 793; Khemani, *Canadian Group Insurance Benefits*, 7-1.
15 Peter Milgram, *Regulation and the Quality of Dental Care* (Germantown, MD: Aspen Systems Corporation, 1978), 153.

16 Khemani, *Canadian Group Insurance Benefits*, 7-2.

17 Deric Johnson, "Employer Experience: Case Study No. 1," in Conference Board of Canada, *Dental Plans in Canada: Growing Employee Benefit* (Ottawa: Conference Board of Canada, 1977), 68.

18 Conference Board of Canada, *Dental Plans in Canada: Growing Employee Benefit* (Ottawa: Conference Board of Canada, 1977). For more on the rapid growth of dental insurance in the 1970s, see Clayton Sinclair, "Canadian Dental Insurance Industry Prospers," *Calgary Herald*, 3 April 1978, A20. An article in *Benefits Canada* claimed that three million Canadians had access to dental insurance in 1976. Darryl Leach and Peter Hirst, "A Dental Discourse," *Benefits Canada* 10, no. 4 (April 1986): 51.

19 Conference Board of Canada, *Dental Plans in Canada*, 2.

20 Stamm et al., *Dental Care Programs in Canada*, 95, 99.

21 Ibid., 100.

22 Peter C. Hirst, "Rapid Dental Plan Growth Slows, But Benefits Improve," *Globe and Mail*, 24 Aug. 1984, S5.

23 *Report on the Findings*, 11; "ABC's Compensation in the Nineties," *Benefits Canada* 14, no. 1 (Jan.–Feb. 1990): 23; Darryl Leach and Peter Hirst, "A Dental Discourse," *Benefits Canada* 10, no. 4 (April 1986): 51.

24 Chanel Ramraj, Laleh Sadeghi, Herenia P. Lawrence, Laura Dempster, and Carlos Quiñonez, "Is Accessing Dental Care Becoming More Difficult? Evidence from Canada's Middle Income Population," *PLOS One* 8, no. 2 (Feb. 2013): 1.

25 *Report on the Findings*, 11.

26 A.M. Hunt, D.W. Lewish, and D.W. Banting, *A Study of Dental Manpower Systems in Relation to Oral Health Status Part 1: Final Report* (Toronto, 1978), 502.

27 Lawrence Welsh, "Dentists' Fee Setting Held Group Plan Threat," *Globe and Mail*, 20 June 1975, B3.

28 Lawrence Welsh, "Group Dental Insurance Plan Is Canada's Most Popular Benefit," *Globe and Mail*, 15 April 1978, B1.

29 "Class-Oriented Cosmetic Service," *Globe and Mail*, 20 May 1969, 12.

30 Ibid., 12.

31 Pay Research Bureau, *Employee Benefits and Working Conditions, Canada 1980* (Ottawa, 1981), 48.

32 *Report on the Findings*, 70.

33 "Measuring the Benefits Equity Gap," *Benefits Canada* 18, no. 8 (Sept. 1994): 13.

34 *Report on the Findings*, 70.

35 Robert G. Evans, "Old Bones, New Data: Emmett Hall, Private Insurance and the Defeat of Pharmacare," *Health Policy* 4, no. 3 (Feb. 2009): 16–24; Robert G. Evans, "Raising the Money: Options, Consequences and Objectives

for Financing Health Care in Canada," *Discussion Paper No. 27, Commission on the Future of Health Care in Canada*, 8, https://pdfs.semanticscholar.org/6dda/74129bd381f8ef1f6d1a945803c00f352c03.pdf <2 Sept. 2021>.

36 Evans, "Raising the Money," 8.

37 Hirst, "Rapid Dental Plan," s5.

38 Conference Board of Canada, *Dental Plans in Canada*, 103–4.

39 Hirst, "Rapid Dental Plan," s5.

40 David Kagan, "Biting Changes," *Benefits Canada* 13, no. 5 (May 1989): 3–5.

41 Ibid., 3–5.

42 Edward Clifford, "Insurance Offering Reduced Benefits in Dental Plans," *Globe and Mail*, 24 Dec. 1993, B3.

43 Sandra Dudley, "Clamping Down on Claims Assignment," *Benefits Canada* 12, no. 11 (Nov. 1988): 30.

44 Ibid., 31.

45 Angela Barnes, "London Life Set for Long Pull with New Pre-paid Dental Plan," *Globe and Mail*, 13 May 1986, B8.

46 Carol Bruman, "Department Store Dentistry," *Maclean's*, 14 Sept. 1981, n.p.; Tasmin Carlisle, "Tridont Keeps on Growing As Its Profits Hit Record," *Globe and Mail*, 23 Sept. 1987, B3; Joan Breckinridge, "Storefront Dentistry Becomes $40 Million Business," *Globe and Mail*, 24 Sept. 1984, B8.

47 "Department-store Dentistry Eliminates Inconvenience," *Calgary Herald*, 8 Aug. 1980, D1.

48 Christopher Donville, "Prepaid Dental Plans Steadily Gain Ground," *Globe and Mail*, 10 July 1987, B17.

49 Marina Strauss, "Prepaid Plans: Will Dentists Bite?" *Globe and Mail*, 9 Feb. 1987, B1.

50 Eric Roher, "Dentists Say New Insurance Plan May Reduce Quality of Treatment," *Globe and Mail*, 1 Sept. 1986, A10.

51 Philippa Dean, "Provincial Union Considers Its Own Denticare Program," *Benefits Canada* 1, no. 8 (Sept.–Oct. 1977): 43–4.

52 Joan Wier-Murrell, "Dental Exposure," *Benefits Canada* 22, no. 3 (March 1998): 47–50. A review of capitation programs can be found in "Capitation's Spreading Roots," *Benefits Canada* 12, no. 4 (April 1988): 27–30.

53 Julie Charles, "Health Benefits: Here and Now," *Benefits Canada* 18, no. 19 (Nov. 1994): 27–31. A survey done the year before found that 79 per cent of employers with benefits were planning to increase deductibles, reduce coverage, or modify the cost-sharing formula to reduce costs. Victor Pywowarczuk, "School's in on Flex Plans," *Benefits Canada* 18, no. 8 (Sept. 1994): 47–9.

54 Charles, "Health Benefits: Here and Now," 27–31.

55 Alex Harvey and Bill Scott, "Claims Busters," *Benefits Canada* 17, no. 1 (Jan. 1993): 32–3.

56 Pywowarczuk, "School's In on Flex Plans," 47–9.
57 Gerald Leavens, "Dental Plan Check-up," *Benefits Canada* 26, no. 1 (Jan. 2002): 31–2.
58 Marg French and David Kogan, "Open Wide," *Benefits Canada* 30, no. 2 (Feb. 2006): 37.
59 Christopher Clark, "Are Dentists Overtreating Their Patients?," *JCDA* 64 (1998): 773-4.
60 Ibid., 773–4.
61 French and Kogon, "Open Wide," 37.
62 Christiane Bourassa and Fern WhitehousKog, "Does Your Dental Plan Need a Check-up?," *Benefits Canada* 27, no. 4 (April 2003): 70–3.
63 Clark, "Are Dentists Overtreating?," 773–4.
64 Jack Pilchar, "Biting Back," *Benefits Canada* 20, no. 6 (June 1996): 13.
65 Jack Pilchar, "Like Pulling Teeth," *Benefits Canada* 21, no. 8 (Sept. 1997): 57–8.
66 Evans, "Raising the Money," 7.
67 Barrie McKenna, "Taxation of Health, Dental Benefit Plans Assailed," *Globe and Mail*, 9 Nov. 1994, B1; Jane Coutts, "Better Oral Health Changes Face of Dentistry," *Globe and Mail*, 21 Feb. 1995, A6.
68 Margot Gibb-Clark, "Quebec's Benefits Tax Leads to Dropouts," *Globe and Mail*, 6 Jan. 1995, B10.
69 Amy Finelstein, "The Effect of Tax Subsidies to Employer-Provided Supplementary Health Insurance: Evidence from Canada," *Journal of Public Economics* 84 (2002): 305–30.
70 CDA ad, "Enough Is Enough," *Globe and Mail*, 11 Jan. 1995, A7.
71 Patricia Surtel, Melissa Philipps, and Charlene Milton, "Emerging Issues," *Benefits Canada* 20, no. 3 (March 1996): 51.
72 April Scott-Clarke, "Scaling Back?" *Benefits Canada* 33, no. 2 (Feb. 2009): 30–2.
73 French and Kogan, "Open Wide," 37; Rosemary Person, "Brushing Up," *Benefits Canada* 31, no. 4 (April 2007): 77.
74 Chantel Ramraj et al., "A Macroeconomic Review of Dentistry in Canada in the 2000s," *JCDA* 80, no. 55 (2014): 1–6. During the 2000s, per-capita spending on dentistry per year increased from $233.94 to $327.84 (in constant dollars), but the amount covered by private dental insurance dropped from $184 per insured person to $145 (in constant dollars.)
75 Wayne J. Millar and David Locker, "Dental Insurance and Use of Dental Services," *Health Reports* 11, no. 1 (1999), 59.
76 In Ontario, among people in Toronto, North York, Simcoe County, and Sudbury and District aged 50–64, 62.1 per cent had insurance, but only 16.7 per cent of those over 75. David Locker and James L. Leake, "Inequities in Health: Dental Insurance Coverage and Use of Dental Services among Older Ontario Adults," *Canadian Journal of Public Health* 84, no. 2 (1993): 139–40.
77 Ibid., 139–40.

78 In Quebec, 78.4 per cent of insured people had visited a dentist in the previous year, but only 60.7 per cent of those without. Jean-Marc Brodeur et al., *Étude 1994–5 sur la santé buccodentaire des adultes québécois de 35 à 44 ans* (Quebec, 1998), 3.
79 Millar and Locker, "Dental Insurance," 60.
80 Among young adults (20–39 years old), 14.1 per cent of the privately insured reported fair or poor oral health, compared to 23.3 per cent of the uninsured. Among adults (40–59), 14.8 per cent of the privately insured reported fair or poor oral health, and 20.6 per cent of the uninsured. *Oral Health Measures Survey* (Ottawa: Health Canada, 2010), 71, https://publications.gc.ca/site/eng/369649/publication.html <30 Sept. 2021>. The privately insured were also far more likely than the uninsured to have visited a dentist – among young adults, 75 per cent versus only 53 per cent, respectively; among adults, 85.4 per cent compared to 57.7 per cent, respectively. *Oral Health Measures Survey*, 77.
81 "The Children Who Dare Not Smile," *Toronto Star*, 4 May 1979, C4.
82 Carlos Quiñonez and Rafael Figueirdo, "Sorry, Doctor, I Can't Afford the Root Canal, I Have a Job: Canadian Dental Care Policy and the Working Poor," *Canadian Journal of Public Health* (Nov.–Dec. 2010): 481–5.
83 Barbara Yaffe, "Drill, Fill and Bill," *Globe and Mail*, 16 July 1979, 4.
84 Ibid., 4.
85 Sasha Mullally and David Wright, *Foreign Practices: Immigrant Doctors and the History of Canadian Medicare* (Montreal: McGill-Queen's University Press, 2020), 78–83.
86 Catherine Carstairs and Ian Mosby, "Colonial Extractions: Oral Health Care and Indigenous People in Canada, 1945–1979," *Canadian Historical Review* 101, no. 2 (June 2020): 192–216.
87 Ian Mosby and Catherine Carstairs, "Federal Policies Undermine Indigenous Dental Health," *Policy Options* 5, Oct. 2018, https://policyoptions.irpp.org/magazines/october-2018/federal-policies-undermine-indigenous-dental-health/ <2 Sept. 2021>.
88 "Survey of Dentists in Canada," *JCDA* 14, no. 2 (Feb. 1948): 45.
89 Canadian Dental Association, *Brief Submitted to the Royal Commission on Health Services by the Canadian Dental Association* (Toronto: Canadian Dental Association, 1962), 15.
90 Douglas Collins, "Finding Dentists Like Pulling Teeth," *Globe and Mail*, 29 July 1957, 6.
91 Canadian Dental Association, *Brief Submitted to the Royal Commission*, VI-5.
92 Task Force on Dental Care, *Interim Report: A Report of the Nova Scotia Council on Health* (Halifax, 1972), 11.
93 Interview with Mary Pelletier, 13 Jan. 2016.
94 Andrew Snaddon, "Alberta Puts Teeth into Plan," *Globe and Mail*, 7 Dec. 1959, 7.
95 Ian Montagnes, "This Town Has No Dentist," *Globe and Mail*, 7 June 1962, 7.

96 Ibid.
97 "Canadian Dental Association News," *JCDA*, 16, no. 3 (March 1950): 152.
98 Canadian Dental Association, *Brief Submitted to the Royal Commission*, VI-3.
99 "A Message from the Dean," *Hya Yaka* (1958–59), 5–7.
100. "Top Dentist Graduate Says Medical Knowledge Needed," *Vancouver Sun*, 24 May 1969, 40.
101 Health Information Division, Policy and Consultation Branch, *Health Personnel in Canada 1992* (Ottawa: Minister of Supply and Services Canada, 1995), 46; *Canada Health Manpower Inventory 1973*, 16.
102 Bruce McFarlane, *Dental Manpower in Canada* (Ottawa, 1965), 17.
103 Ibid., 19.
104 "Support for Dental Surgeon's Plea," *Saskatoon Star Phoenix*, 18 March 1960, 17.
105 "Dental Board of Governors Approve Recruiting Plan," *Saskatoon Star Phoenix*, 2 June 1961, 2.
106 Canadian Dental Association, *Survey of Dental Practice 1963* (Toronto: Canadian Dental Association, 1963), 7.
107 "Average Income of Canadian Dentists," *JCDA* 27, no. 12 (Dec. 1961): 797.
108 Ibid., 798. Between 1949 and 1959, dentists' average incomes had increased by 102 per cent, physicians and surgeons' by 75 per cent, and engineers and architects' by 44 per cent. Overall, average incomes had grown by 43 per cent.
109 "Survey Shows Dentists Favour Recruitment," *JCDA* 27, no. 12 (Dec. 1961): 799–807.
110 The biggest jump in applicants occurred in the early 1970s. Canadian Dental Association, *Applicants and Applications to Canadian Dental Schools*. This was a serial produced 1966–75.
111 Yaffe, "Drill, Fill and Bill," 4. In 1965–66, it was harder to get into dental than medical schools, although more people made multiple applications, which suggests that they did not realize this. D.G. Fish and B. Isabel Brown, "A Comparison of Applicants and Applications to Canadian Medical and Dental Schools," *Canadian Medical Association Journal* 95, no. 2 (9 July 1996): 68–71.
112 Fish and Brown, "A Comparison," 68–71.
113 "Student Recruitment Should Emphasize Quality," *JCDA* 31, no. 5 (May 1965): 338–9.
114 H.K. Brown, "The Need for Dental Services in Rural Areas," *JCDA* 27, no. 6 (June 1961): 367.
115 C.H. McCormick, "Availability and Utilization of Dental Services by Rural Manitoba Children," *JCDA* 32, no. 3 (1966): 251.
116 *Final Report of the Advisory Planning Committee on Medical Care to the Government of Saskatchewan* (Saskatoon, 1962), 75; "In Rural Dentistry," *Globe and Mail*, 12 May 1965, 5.
117 Canadian Dental Association, *Survey of Dental Practice 1963*, 9.
118 *Final Report of the Advisory Planning Committee*, 75.

119 "How Are You Going to Keep 'Em Down on the Farm?," *JCDA* 39, no. 3 (March 1974): 167.
120 "CDA Committee Report: Applicants to Canadian [*sic*] Dental Schools 1982–3: Who Are They? What Are They Like?," *JCDA* 49, 1 (Jan. 1984): 57–62.
121 Leslie Robinson, "Dental Public Health Programs for the Province of British Columbia," *JCDA* 17, no. 6 (June 1951): 314.
122 Task Force on Dental Care, *Final Report: A Report to the Nova Scotia Council on Health* (Halifax, 1973), 44. Quebec's program was apparently not very robust. Ibid., 80.
123 C.H. McCormick, "Dentists' Suggestions for Improving Dental Care in Rural Manitoba," *JCDA* 34, no. 10 (Oct. 1968): 533.
124 "Prince Edward Island Increases Dental Student Aid," *JCDA* 35, no. 6 (June 1969): 293.
125 Barbara Yaffe, "Tooth Trouble: A Painful Look at the State of Canada's Dental Health," *Globe and Mail*, 14 July 1979, P1.
126 *Final Report of the Advisory Planning Committee*, 82.
127 R.E. McDermott and J.J. Tynan, "Attracting Dental Graduates to Rural Locations: Evaluation of the Saskatchewan Initiative," *Canadian Journal of Community Dentistry* 3, no. 2 (1986): 25.
128 Task Force on Dental Care, *Final Report*, 44.
129 Nova Scotia Dental Association, *83rd Annual Report*, June 1973, 10.
130 Nova Scotia Dental Association, *84th Annual Report*, June 1974, 15-3.
131 "Too Few Apply for Bursaries, Dentist Says," *Globe and Mail*, 22 May 1963, 8.
132 Bill Prager, "Sixteen Doctors Skip Conditions," *Windsor Star*, 26 April 1973, 32.
133 Mary Golem, "Dentist Brightening Smiles for over Forty Years," *Sun Times* (Owen Sound), 29 Jan. 2008, B1.
134 Joan Hollobon, "Dentists Strive to Fill Gaps," *Globe and Mail*, 6 April 1961, 25.
135 "Program Set to Attract Dentists to Rural Areas of Province," *Saskatoon Star Phoenix*, 19 July 1966, 3.
136 "Dentists Enticed," *Gazette*, 10 July 1975, 21; "Dentist Shortage Said Improving," *Saskatoon Star Phoenix*, 17 July 1976, 24.
137 Mullally and Wright, *Foreign Practices*, 52–6.
138 N.H.F. Wilson and S. Gelbier, "Dental Witness Seminars: Dentistry in the UK since 1994," *British Dental Journal* 220, no. 3 (2016), 135.
139 *Final Report of the Advisory Planning Committee*, 90.
140 Task Force on Dental Care, *Final Report*, 21–2.
141 Ibid., 22.
142 "'Quality of Care' behind Immigrant Doctor Rule," *Vancouver Sun*, 11 May 1976, 8.
143 Joanne Munro, "Mobile Dental Clinic," *Edmonton Journal*, 19 Dec. 1979, 41; John I. Woronuk et al., "University of Alberta Dental Students Outreach

Clinical Experience: An Evaluation of the Program," *JCDA* 70, no. 4 (April 2004): 233–6.

144 H.K. Brown, "The Need for Dental Services in Rural Areas," *JCDA* 27, no. 6 (June 1961): 367. "Whistlestop Dentist: Car Covers Northern Ontario," *Ottawa Citizen*, 1 Aug. 1951, 3.

145 Melville Germa, MPP, Ontario Hansard, Session 31: 1, Thursday 7 July 1977.

146 Sasha Mullally and David Wright, "La grande séduction," *Journal of Canadian Studies* 41, no. 3 (2007): 67–89; William S. Hacon, "Health Manpower in Canada," *Canadian Journal of Public Health* 64, no. 1 (1973): 10–11.

147 Gilles Dussault, "Dental Services in Quebec: Issues and Changes," *Social Science and Medicine* 18, no. 3 (1984): 252.

148 "Stream of New Dentists Flooding Market, Say Established Professionals," *Calgary Herald*, 21 Sept. 1979, 22.

149 Deanna Herman, "Dentists Needed in Rural Areas," *Saskatoon Star Phoenix*, 10 Dec. 1987, 3.

150 Millar and Locker, "Dental Insurance," 57. In 1996–97, 46 per cent of rural Canadians and 54 per cent of urban residents had dental coverage.

151 Bill Shields, "Two-Car Families on the Increase," *Windsor Star*, 29 June 1973, 32; Joyce Dargay and Dermot Gatley, "Income's Effects on Car and Vehicle Ownership, Worldwide: 1960–2015," *Transportation Research Part A: Policy and Practice* 33, no. 2 (1999): 101–38.

152 "Gravelbourg Can't Get Dentist after Province Axes Therapist," *Saskatoon Star Phoenix*, 19 Dec. 1987, 7.

153 "Dental Therapists Ask Right to Establish Rural Offices," *Saskatoon Star Phoenix*, 3 Feb. 1988, 3.

154 McDermott and Tynan, "Attracting Dental Graduates," 24–8.

155 Jan Wong, "Fluoride Has Dentists Frowning," *Globe and Mail*, 21 March 1996, A1.

156 D.V. Parmenter, "Dental Manpower: An Atlantic Perspective," *JCDA* 52, no. 1 (1986): 65.

157 Norman Provencher, "Surplus of Dentists Could Grow," *Globe and Mail*, 10 Sept. 1982, R1.

158 "N.W.T. Requires Dentists Urgently," *JCDA* 35, no. 3 (March 1980): 158.

159 Nastaran Sharifan et al., "Dental Students' Perspectives on Rural Dental Practice: A Qualitative Study," *JCDA* 81 (2 Dec. 2015): f23, https://jcda.ca/article/f23 <3 Sept. 2021>.

160 Ibid., f23.

161 Gil McGowan, "Alarm Raised over Shortage of Dentists in Rural Alberta," *Edmonton Journal*, 13 June 1994, C12.

162 Elham Emani et al., "Oral Health and Access to Dental Care: A Qualitative Exploration in Rural Quebec," *Canadian Journal of Rural Medicine* 19, no. 2 (2014): 64.

163 E. Emani et al., "Mapping the Quebec Dental Workforce: Ranking Rural Oral Health Disparities," *Rural and Remote Health* 16 (2016), n.p.
164 Emani et al., "Oral Health and Access to Dental Care," 63–70.
165 Amal Gaber et al., "Rural–Urban Disparity in Oral Health–Related Quality of Life," *Community Dentistry and Oral Epidemiology* 46 (2017): 132–42.
166 Julie Kosteniuk, "Dental Service Use and Its Correlates in a Dentate Population: An Analysis of the Saskatchewan Population Health and Dynamics Survey, 1999-2000," *JCDA* 72, no. 8 (2006): 731a.
167 Robert J. Schroth et al., "Trends in Pediatric Dental Surgery for Severe Early Childhood Caries in Manitoba," *JCDA* 80, no. 65 (25 Nov. 2014): n.p., https://jcda.ca/article/e65 <3 Sept. 2021>.
168 Jack Lee, "A Comparison of the Dental Health of Toronto's Ethnic Groups," *Canadian Journal of Community Dentistry* 2, no. 2 (July 1987): 8–9.
169 Graham L. Woodward and James L. Leake, "Risk Markers for New Dental Decay in Eight-Year-Old North York Children," *Canadian Journal of Community Dentistry* 10, no. 2 (Sept. 1985): 10.
170 Renata I. Werneck et al., "Early Childhood Caries and Access to Dental Care among Children of Portuguese Speaking Immigrants in the City of Toronto," *JCDA* 74, no. 9 (2008): 805.
171 Werneck et al., "Early Childhood Caries," 805.
172 Jeffrey G. Reitz and Anil Verma, "Immigration, Race and Labor: Unionization and Wages in the Canadian Labour Market," *Industrial Relations* 43, no. 4 (Oct. 2004): 835–54.
173 James Ted McDonald and Steven Kennedy, "Insights into the 'Healthy Immigrant Effect': Health Status and Health Service Use of Immigrants to Canada," *Social Science and Medicine* 59, no. 8 (Oct. 2004): 1613–27.
174 K. Bruce Newbold and Amish Patel, "Use of Dental Services by Immigrant Canadians," *JCDA* 72, no. 3 (March 2006): 143.
175 Ibid., 143.
176 P. Calvasina et al., "The Deterioration of Canadian Immigrants' Oral Health: An Analysis of the Longitudinal Survey of Immigrants to Canada," *Community Dentistry and Oral Epidemiology* 43 (2015): 424–32.
177 Paola Calvasina, Carles Muntaner, and Carlos Quiñonez, "Factors Associated with Unmet Dental Care Needs in Canadian Immigrants," *BMC Oral Health* 14 (2014): 145.
178 Maryan S. Amin et al., "Parental Awareness and Dental Attendance of Children among African Immigrants," *Journal of Immigrant and Minority Health* 17 (2015): 132–8.
179 Edmond Ghiabi, Debora C. Matthews, and Martha Smith Brillant, "The Oral Health Status of Recent Immigrants and Refugees," *Journal of Immigrant and Minority Health* 16 (2014), 95–101.
180 Daniel W.L. Lai and Nelson T.A. Hui, "Use of Dental Care by Elderly Chinese

Immigrants in Canada," *Journal of Public Health Dentistry* 67, no. 1 (2007): 56–9.

181 Michael I. MacEntee et al., "Discussions on Oral Health Care among Elderly Chinese Immigrants in Melbourne and Vancouver," *Gerondontology* 29 (2012): 8e22–32.

182 Mei Dong et al., "Chinese Immigrants' Dental Care Pathways in Montreal Canada," *JCDA* 77 (2011): b131.

183 K.M. Nasir, "An Immigrant's Struggles in Canada," 26 May 2011, https://canadianimmigrant.ca/living/community/an-immigrants-struggles-in-canada <3 Sept. 2021>.

184 Paolo Calvasina, Herenia P. Lawrence, Laurie Hoffman-Goetz, and Cameron D. Norman, "Brazilian Immigrants' Oral Health Literacy and Participation in Oral Health Care in Canada," *BMC Oral Health* 16, (2016): 18.

185 P. Calvasina, P. Muntaner, and C. Quiñonez, "Transnational Dental Care among Canadian Immigrants," *Community Dentistry and Oral Epidemiology* 43 (2015): 441–51.

186 "Taking a Bite out of Inequality: Universal Dentalcare for Canada," 19 Jan. 2021, https://www.youtube.com/watch?v=iWVHSyNtCDk <3 Sept. 2021>.

187 Carlos Quiñonez, "Self-Reported Emergency Room Visits for Dental Problems," *International Journal of Dental Hygiene* 9 (2011): 17–20.

188 Carlos Quiñonez, Debbie Gibson, Aleksandra Jokovic, and David Locker, "Emergency Department Visits for Dental Care of Nontraumatic Origin," *Community Dentistry and Oral Epidemiology* 37, no. 4 (2009): 366–71.

189 Sonica Singhal, Lindsay McLaren, and Carlos Quiñonez "Trends in Emergency Department Visits for Non-traumatic Dental Conditions in Ontario from 2006–2014," *Canadian Journal of Public Health* 108 (2017): e246–50.

190 Mario Brondani and Syed H. Ahmand "The 1% of Emergency Room Visits for Non-traumatic Dental Conditions in British Columbia: Misconceptions about the Numbers," *Canadian Journal of Public Health* 108 (2017): e279–81.

Chapter Five

1 Nadine Jones, "Important to Get a Grip on Denture Issues: Quick Repairs with Crazy Glue Thankfully Past," *Vancouver Sun*, 8 Aug. 1994, C5. Another article on Jones indicates that she must have been born about 1924. (In 2015, she reports being 91.) Nadine Jones, "Nadina, 91, Decided It Was Time to Move," *Richmond News*, 23 Oct. 2015, http://www.richmond-news.com/news/weekly-feature/nadine-91-decided-it-was-time-to-move-1.2094071 <4 Sept. 2021>.

2 M. Straker and I.B. Hyams, "Some Psychological Implications of Dental Practice," *JCDA* 16, no. 7 (July 1950): 355–9.

3 Patient quoted in Sanford Plainfield, "Psychological Considerations in Prosthetic Dentistry," in Loren R. Borland and Paul Wesley Vinton, eds,

Dental Clinics of North America: Symposium on I. Psychology in Dentistry and II. Removable Partial Dentures (Philadelphia and London: W.B. Saunders and Company, 1962), 671.

4 Michael MacEntee, Rachelle Hole, and Elaine Stoler, "The Significance of the Mouth in Old Age," *Social Science Medicine* 45, no. 9 (1997): 1453.

5 Ontario, *A Smile for All Seasons: Facts about Dentures*, pamphlet, Ministry of Health, 1980; Polident advertisements in the 1940s warned about the horrors of "denture breath": "False Teeth Wearers How Awful – Denture Breath," *Life Magazine* (1946), http://library.duke.edu/digitalcollections/mma_MM0112/ <4 Sept. 2021>; "False Teeth Wearers Often the Worst Breath Offenders," *Better Home and Gardens* (1941), http://library.duke.edu/digitalcollections/mma_MM0111/ <4 Sept. 2021>; Mia Stainsby, "Dental Implants Give Snugger Fit," *Vancouver Sun*, 16 April 2001, B8; Meyer M. Silverman, "Pre-Extraction Records to Avoid Premature Aging of the Denture Patient," JCDA 21, no. 9 (Sept. 1955): 522–3; Malcolm Yasny, "New Dentures Can Ease Wrinkles," *Toronto Star*, 11 Oct. 1986, F4; Malcolm Yasny, "Depressed Dental Patients Need Some Psychiatric Help," *Toronto Star*, 15 Oct. 1988, G2; John S. Anderson and Roy Storer, *Immediate and Replacement Dentures* (Oxford: Blackwell Scientific Publications, 1973); Carl O. Flagstad, "Problems in Denture Services," JCDA 12, no. 2 (Feb. 1946): 75–6.

6 Simone de Beauvoir, *The Coming of Age* (New York: Putnam, 1972); Laura Herd Clarke, *Facing Age: Women Growing Older in Anti-Aging Culture* (Lanham, MD: Rowman and Littlefield, 2011).

7 Frank Furniss, "An Essay on Denture Practice," JCDA 15, no. 4 (April 1949): 215–16.

8 R.O. Schlosser, "The Significance of Balanced Occlusion within and beyond the Normal Functional Range in Complete Denture Prosthesis," JCDA 16, no. 2 (Feb. 1950): 67–74; D.V. Lloyd, "Full Dentures Using Natural Teeth," JCDA 16, no. 7 (July 1950): 353–5; M. Straker and I.B. Hyams, "Some Psychological Implications of Dental Practice," JCDA 16, no. 7 (July 1950): 355–9; Howard J. Merkely, "That Flat Lower Again," JCDA 18, no. 2 (Feb. 1952): 73; Howard Merkeley, "Assisting Patients with Dental Prosthesis," JCDA 19, no. 1 (Jan. 1953): 11–13; A.H. Schmidt, "Planning and Designing Removable Partial Dentures," JCDA 20, no. 8 (Aug. 1954): 415; H.H. Pearson, "Oral Facial and Mental Rehabilitation," JCDA 24, no. 9 (Sept. 1958): 597–8.

9 "Dental Care for Senior Citizens," JCDA 31, no. 2 (Feb. 1965): 124.

10 M.I. MacEntee and M.F. Williamson, "Attitudes of Dentists in British Columbia to Dental Technicians, Dental Mechanics and Removable Prosthodontics," JCDA 46, no. 12 (Dec. 1980): 768–71.

11 Carl O. Boucher, Judson C. Hickey, and George A. Zarb, *Prosthodontic Treatment for Edentulous Patients* (St Louis, MO: C.V. Mosby, 1975), 17–18; John Osborne and George Alexander Lammie, *Partial Dentures* (Oxford: Oxford Scientific Publications, 1968), 18–23; John H. Wilson, *Partial Dentures: A*

Manual for Students and Practitioners of Dentistry (Philadelphia: Lea and Febiger, 1957), 83–4.

12 A.M. Hunt, D.W. Lewis, and D.W. Banting, *A Study of Dental Manpower Systems in Relation to Oral Health Status, Part I: Ontario* (Toronto: Faculty of Dentistry, 1978), 23–4.

13 Byron S. Hollinshead, *The Survey of Dentistry: The Final Report* (Washington, DC: American Council on Education, 1961), 26.

14 Tracey L. Adams, *A Dentist and a Gentleman: Gender and the Rise of Dentistry in Ontario* (Toronto: University of Toronto Press, 2000), 70.

15 By 1970, there were dental-technician programs at the Édouard Montpetit CÉGEP in Longueuil, Quebec, the George Brown College of Applied Arts and Technology in Toronto, the Northern Albert Institute of Technology in Edmonton, and the Vancouver Vocational Institute. *Ad Hoc Committee on Dental Auxiliaries* (Ottawa: Information Canada, 1970), 35.

16 Joan Boase, "Regulation and the Paramedical Professions: An Interest Group Study," *Canadian Public Administration / Administration publique du Canada* 25, no. 3 (autumn 1982): 332–53; David Coburn, "Professionalization and Proletarianization: Medicine, Nursing and Chiropractic in Historical Perspective," *Labour / Le Travail* 34 (autumn 1994): 139–62.

17 Warren Gerard, "Denturist Feud Leaves Public in the Middle," *Toronto Star*, 23 Jan. 1974, B3.

18 Ibid.

19 "Dentists to Pay for Her Teeth," *Toronto Star*, 12 Jan. 1974, A1.

20 Bruce A. McFarlane, *Dental Manpower in Canada* (Ottawa: Queen's Printer, 1965), 163–70.

21 J.W. Neilson, "Manpower in Dentistry: The Dental Technician," *JCDA* 27, no. 1 (Jan. 1961): 13.

22 Ibid., 13–18.

23 Alan D. Fee, "The Dental Mechanics of Canada," *Journal of Prosthetic Dentistry* 31, no. 1 (Jan. 1974): 12; Barbara Himmel, *Denturists: The Birth of a Profession* (Sherwood Park: Denturist Society of Alberta, 1986), 23–9.

24 Himmel, *Denturists*, 14–15.

25 Fee, "The Dental Mechanics," 13–14.

26 G.C. Swann, "The Next Step," *JCDA* 27, no. 4 (April 1961): 644–6.

27 Task Force on Dental Care, *Final Report: A Report to the Nova Scotia Council on Health* (Halifax, 1973), 52.

28 "Auxiliary Services," *JCDA* 20, no. 6 (June 1954): 340–3.

29 Fee, "The Dental Mechanics," 13; Himmel, *Denturists*, 117–18.

30 Fee, "The Dental Mechanics," 13.

31 "Journal des débats de la Commission permanent des corporations professionnelles," http://www.assnat.qc.ca/fr/travaux-parlementaires/

commissions/ccp-2-avant-1984-29-4/journal-debats/CCP-730621.html <4 Sept. 2021>.

32 "Aux membres de l'Association des Techniciens dentaires du Québec," *La Presse*, 6 June 1974, 7.
33 "Prosthèses dentaires : Qui est le véritable expert?," *La Presse*, 30 June 1996, C2.
34 Barbara Frum, "The High Cost of Dentures," *Toronto Star*, 18 June 1966, 9.
35 N. John Adams, "Two More Denture Technicians Raided by OPP, College of Dental Surgeons," *Globe and Mail*, 7 May 1971, 8.
36 "End Dentists' Monopoly," *Globe and Mail*, 8 May 1971, 8.
37 "Look First at the Old," *Globe and Mail*, 16 May 1972, 6.
38 "Ontario Will Legalize Denturists' Clinics, Establish a Board to Set Basic Standards," *Globe and Mail*, 27 June 1972, 1–2.
39 Ontario Council of Health, *Report of the Ontario Council of Health Task Force on Dental Technicians*, March 1972.
40 "Denturists Can Continue to Work with the Public up to a Year," *Toronto Star*, 12 Dec. 1972, 28.
41 "Denturists Vow to Defy Law, Risk Jail," *Toronto Star*, 8 Jan. 1973, 34.
42 Sally Barnes, "Anti-denturist Law Might Be Scrapped," *Toronto Star*, 1 June 1973, 3.
43 "Potter Set to Implement Law to Stop Denturists," *Toronto Star*, 28 June 1973, 18.
44 "Room for Compromise with Denturists," *Toronto* Star, 19 Nov. 1973, C4.
45 "Police Stage Two More Denture Clinic Raids," *Toronto Star*, 10 Jan. 1974, B2; "Seven Metro Denturists Charged after Raids," *Toronto Star*, 16 Feb. 1974, A6; "Dental Technician Fined for Practicing without a License," *Toronto Star*, 13 Dec. 1974, B2.
46 "Welch Refused to Drop Denturist Charges," *Toronto Star*, 17 May 1974, A4.
47 Robert Sutton, "Denturists behind Bars Fight on," *Toronto Star*, 31 March 1980, A3.
48 Himmel, *Denturists*, 130.
49 Wayne J. Millar and David Locker, "Edentulism and Denture Use," *Health Reports* 17, no. 1 (Nov. 2005): 56.
50 Kalyani K. Baldota and James L. Leake, "A Macroeconomic Review of Dentistry in Canada in the 1990s," *JCDA* 70, no. 9 (Sept. 2004): 604–9.
51 "Absolutely Dentures," http://www.absolutelydentures.com/why-choose-denturist/, <11 May 2020>; "Bajic Dental Clinic," https://www.bajicdentures.ca/should-you-choose-a-dentist-or-denturist/, <11 May 2020>; "Calgary Denture Clinic," https://calgarydentureclinic.net/blog/Dentist+or+Denturist+/93 <11 May 2020>.
52 Tracey L. Adams, *Regulating Professions: The Emergence of Professional Regulation in Four Canadian Provinces* (Toronto: University of Toronto Press, 2018), 197–238.

53 Boase, "Regulation and the Paramedical Professions," 332–53.

54 James Struthers, "Framing Aging through the Senate: Canada's Two Senate Reports on Aging, 1963–66 and 2006–9," *Canadian Review of Social Policy* 68, no. 9 (2012–13): 1–9; C.G. Gifford, *Canada's Fighting Seniors* (Toronto: James Lorimer, 1990), 19–42.

55 Gavin J. Andrews, Lori Campbell, Margaret Denton, and Kathy S. McGilton, "Gerontology in Canada: History, Challenges, Research," *Ageing International* 34, no. 136 (2009): 136–53.

56 The JCDA published its first study of the oral health of the aged in 1969: Irwin Lightman, G.W. Thompson, and R.M. Grainger, "Denture Needs of a Group of Toronto Aged," JCDA 35, no. 1 (Jan. 1969): 40–4. A number of others quickly followed: B.P. Martinello and J.L. Leake, "Oral Health Status in the Three London, Ontario Homes for the Aged," JCDA 37, no. 11 (Nov. 1971): 429–32; B.P. Martinello, "Oral Health Assessment of Residents of a Chatham, Ontario Home for the Aged," JCDA 41, 8 (Aug. 1975): 405–9; J.L. Leake and B.P. Martinello, "Oral Health Status of Independent Elderly Persons in London, Ontario," JCDA 38, no. 1 (Jan. 1972): 31–4. The *Canadian Journal of Public Health* (CJPH) started running articles on the subject at roughly the same time. David Banting, "Dental Care for the Aged," CJPH 62, no. 2 (Nov.–Dec. 1971): 503–8; David W. Banting, "A Study of Dental Care Cost, Time and Treatment Requirements of Older Persons in the Community," CJPH 63, no. 6 (Nov.–Dec. 1972): 508–15.

57 Martinello and Leake, "Oral Health Status … London, Ontario."

58 Martinello, "Oral Health Assessment … Chatham, Ontario."

59 James L. Leake, "A Review of Regional Studies on the Dental Health of Older Canadians," *Gerondontology* 7, no. 1 (1998): 11–19.

60 Marie Demers, Jean-Marc Brodeur, Paul Simar, and Roland Vallée, "Problems Associated with Endentulism among the Elderly," JCDA 52, no. 12 (Dec. 1986): 1019–22; Paul L. Simard, Jean-M. Brodeur, Daniel Kandelman, and Yves Lepage, "Prosthetic Status and Needs of the Elderly in Quebec," JCDA 51, no. 1 (Jan. 1985): 79–81; Jean-M. Brodeur, Paul L. Simard, Daniel Kandelman, and Yves Lepage, "Conclusions from a Study on the Oral Health of Quebecers Aged 65 and Over," JCDA 51, no. 11 (Nov. 1985): 817–19.

61 D.W. Lewis, *Research into Dental Manpower in Ontario: A Summary of Concerns and Findings* (Toronto: Department of Community Dentistry, Faculty of Dentistry, 1981).

62 Erwin Lightman, "Geriatric Treatment a 'Crying Need,'" JCDA 48, no. 6 (May 1982): 347.

63 G.W. Myers, "Treatment of the Elderly: Is Help Ahead?," JCDA 48, no. 10 (Oct. 1982): 611.

64 James D.R. Grier, "Grey Power Doesn't Equal Denture Power," JCDA 50, no. 9 (Sept. 1984): 653.

65 M.I. MacEntee, "The Dentist and the Older Patient," *JCDA* 50, no. 9 (Sept. 1984): 675.

66 J.R. Vincent, P. Massicotte, and R.Y. Barolet, "The Teaching of Geriatric Dentistry in Canada," *JCDA* 58, no. 9 (Sept. 1992): 735.

67 James Leake, "The History of Dental Programs for Older Adults," *JCDA* 66, no. 6 (May 2000): 316–19.

68 Stasia Evasuk, "Seniors Need Education on Caring for Teeth, Dentist Says," *Toronto Star*, 16 June 1986, C4.

69 Heather Murray, David Locker, Martha Clark, and Pat Main, *Oral Health Status and Treatment Needs of Older Adults in North York SS* (Toronto: University of Toronto, Faculty of Dentistry, Community Dental Health Services Research Unit, 1997).

70 Michael MacEntee, "Measuring the Impact of Oral Health in Old Age: A Qualitative Reaction to Some Quantitative Views," *Gerondontology* 13, no. 2 (1996): 76–81; Michael MacEntee, Rachel Weiss, Nancy E. Waxier-Morrison, and Brenda J. Morrison, "Opinions of Dentists on the Treatment of Elderly Patients in Long-term Care Facilities," *Journal of Public Health Dentistry* 52, no. 4 (June 1992): 239–44.

71 The high rate of edentulousness in the north might be connected to the region's long-time shortage of dentists. In 1962, the average resident travelled 50–100 miles (80–160 kilometres) to a dentist. "Thousands in Ontario without a Doctor," *Toronto Star*, 3 Nov. 1962, 4.

72 David Locker and Barbara Payne, *Oral Health Status and the Use of Dental Services among Ontarians Aged Fifty Years or Older* (Toronto: Faculty of Dentistry, Community Dental Health Services Research Unit, 1993).

73 Statistics Canada, *Canadian Health Measures Survey 2007–09* (Ottawa, 2009), 70, 78.

74 Christophe Bedos, Christine Loignon, Anne Landry, Paul J. Allison, and Lucie Richard, "How Health Professionals Perceive and Experience Treating People on Social Assistance: A Qualitative Study among Dentists in Montreal, Canada," *BMC Health Services Research* 13 (2013): 464–73; Christophe Bedos, Jean-Marc Brodeur, Alissa Levine, and Lucie Richard, "Perception of Dental Illness among Persons Receiving Public Assistance in Montreal," *American Journal of Public Health* 95, no. 8 (Aug. 2005): 1340–4.

75 Robert D. Krotzer, Herenia P. Lawrence, Joanne B. Clove, and Debora C Matthews, "Oral Health–Related Quality of Life in an Aging Canadian Population," *Health and Quality of Life Outcomes* 10 (2012): 8.

76 Robert H. Binstock, "The Search for Prolongevity: A Contentious Pursuit," in Stephen Garrard and Robert H. Binstock, eds, *The Fountain of Youth: Cultural, Scientific and Ethical Perspectives on a Biomedical Goal* (Oxford: Oxford University Press, 2004), 17–18.

77 Carole Haber, "Anti-Aging: Why Now? A Historical Framework for

Understanding the Contemporary Enthusiasm," *Generations* 25, no. 4 (winter 2001–02): 13.

78 "Interview with Dr. George Zarb," *JCDA* 71, no. 5 (May 2005): 321–3; Tomas Alberktsson and Ann Wennerberg, "The Impact of Oral Implants: Past and Future, 1966–2042," *JCDA* 71, no. 5 (May 2005): 327a–327d.

79 Erla Kay, "The Canadian Implant Institute," *Dental Practice Management* (autumn 1998), 36.

80 A review of the telephone *Yellow Pages* for Toronto shows that in 1993 only eight dentists advertised implants as part of their practice. The city's *Central East Directory* for 2002–03 had 19 dentists doing so.

81 Mia Stainsby, "Dental Implants Give a Snugger Fit," *Trail [BC] Times*, 27 April 2001, 9; Greg Williams, "Dental Implants Bring out the Smiles," *Calgary Herald*, 8 Aug. 2002, s8; "Dental Work: Titanium Implants Give a Snug Fit," *Sault Star*, 21 April 2001, E4; Daniel Nach, "Dental Implants Can Help Bring back Perfect Smile," *Times & Transcript* (Moncton), 7 April 2007, E2; Walter Heidary, "Implants Can Replace Loose Dentures," *Hamilton Spectator*, 10 Sept. 2001, C08.

82 Grania Litwin, "A Better Bite: Dental Implants Can Be an Effective Option for Severe Dental Problems," *Victoria Times Colonist*, 15 June 2001, C5.

83 Litwin, "A Better Bite," C5.

84 Ibid., C5.

85 Veronique Mandal, "Same-day Teeth: Swedish Technology," *Windsor Star*, 21 Feb. 2002, F5.

86 Bjarni E. Pjeturrson, Urs Bragger, Niklaus P. Lang, and Marcel Zwahlen, "Comparisons of Survival and Complication Rates of Tooth Supported Fixed Dental Prostheses (FDPS) and Implant-Supported Prostheses (FDPS) and Single Crowns (SCS)," *Clinical Oral Implants Research* 18 (Suppl. 3) (2007): 97–113.

87 Alberktsson and Wennerberg, "The Impact of Oral Implants," 327a–327d.

88 Michael MacEntee, *The Complete Denture: A Clinical Pathway* (Chicago: Quintessence Publishing, 1999), ix.

89 Don Ihde, "Aging: I Don't Want to Be a Cyborg!" *Phenomenology and the Cognitive Sciences* 7, no. 3 (Sept. 2008): 397–404.

90 Steve Anderson and Walter Hailey, "Stop Losing Patients You Have Never Met," *Dental Practice Management* (summer 1990): 40–1.

91 "Dental Benefits Guide: Non-insured Health Benefits," https://www.sac-isc.gc.ca/eng/1579538771806/1579538804799 <12 May 2020>.

Chapter Six

1 Sara Kettler, "The Story behind Farrah Fawcett's Iconic 1976 Swimsuit Poster," https://www.biography.com/news/farrah-fawcett-swimsuit-poster <12 Oct. 2021>.

2 Joanna Schneller, "What Big, White Choppers Those Actors Have," *Globe and Mail*, 27 Aug. 1999, C1.

3 Elizabeth Haiken, *Venus Envy: A History of Cosmetic Surgery* (Baltimore: John Hopkins University Press, 1997); Kathy Davis, "'A Dubious Equality': Men, Women and Cosmetic Surgery," *Body and Society* 8, no. 1 (2002): 49–65.

4 Norman Wahl, "Orthodontics in Three Millennia. Chapter 1: Antiquity to the Mid-19th Century," *American Journal of Orthodontics and Dentofacial Orthopedics* 127, no. 2 (2005): 255–9.

5 Milton Asbell, "A Brief History of Orthodontics," *American Journal of Orthodontic and Dentofacial Orthopaedics* 98, no. 3 (1998): 206–13; Norman Wahl, "Orthodontics in Three Millennia. Chapter 2: Entering the Modern Era," *American Journal of Orthodontic and Dentofacial Orthopaedics* 127, no. 4 (2005): 510–15.

6 Elizabeth E. Hunt, "How Americans Got Their Straight White Teeth" (PhD diss., University of Pennsylvania, 1998), 180–99.

7 William R. Proffit with Henry W. Fields, *Contemporary Orthodontics*, 2nd ed. (St Louis, MO: Mosby, 1993), 6.

8 Norman Wahl, "Orthodontics in Three Millennia. Chapter 3: The Professionalization of Orthodontics," *Journal of Orthodontics and Dentofacial Orthopedics* 127, no. 6 (2005): 749–53; Norman Wahl, "Orthodontics in Three Millennia. Chapter 11: The Golden Age of Orthodontics," *Journal of Orthodontics and Dentofacial Orthopedics* 130, no. 4 (2006): 549.

9 Jean-Marie Morin, "L'université possède un service renommé," *La Presse*, 6 Feb. 1947, n.p.

10 Canada, *Canada Health Manpower Inventory* (Ottawa: Health and Welfare Canada, 1985), 53; Statistics Canada, Annual Estimates of Population of Canada, by Provinces, http://www.stats.gov.nl.ca/statistics/population/PDF/Annual_Pop_Prov.PDF <5 Sept. 2021>.

11 Haiken, *Venus Envy*, 7, 19; Kathy Peiss, *Hope in a Jar: The Making of America's Beauty Culture* (New York: Metropolitan Books, 1998), 97–133; Jane Nicholas, *The Modern Girl: Feminine Modernities, the Body and Commodities in the 1920s* (Toronto: University of Toronto Press, 2015).

12 Mary Otto, *Teeth: The Story of Beauty, Inequality, and the Struggle for Oral Health in America* (New York: New Press, 2017), 17–18; Ronald Goldstein, *Esthetics in Dentistry*, 2nd ed. (Hamilton, ON, and London: B.C. Decker Inc, 1998), 123; Catherine Exley, "Bridging a Gap: The (Lack of a) Sociology of Oral Health and Healthcare," *Sociology of Health and Illness* 31, no. 7 (2009): 1093–1108. For an excellent article on the growing cultural preference for straight, white teeth, see Abeer Khalid and Carlos Quiñonez, "Straight White Teeth as a Social Prerogative," *Sociology of Health and Illness* 37, no. 5 (2015): 782–96.

13 Fred E.H. Schroeder, "Say Cheese! The Revolution in the Aesthetics of Smiles," *Journal of Popular Culture* 32, no. 2 (Sept. 1998): 103–45. See similar

conclusions in Colin Jones, *The Smile Revolution in Eighteenth Century Paris* (Oxford: Oxford University Press, 2014), 177–84.

14 James McCoy, *Applied Orthodontia* (Philadelphia: Lea & Febiger, 1922), 19–20. McCoy used the same wording in *Applied Orthodontics* (Philadelphia: Lea & Febiger, 1935), 17–18, and in *Applied Orthodontics* (Philadelphia: Lea & Febinger, 1956), 15–17.

15 George M. Anderson, *Practical Orthodontics* (St Louis, MO: C.V. Mosby Company, 1948), 22. The 1960 version said the same on these points. George Anderson, *Practical Orthodontics*, rev. ed. (St Louis, MO: C.V. Mosby Company, 1960), 30.

16 T.M. Graber, *Orthodontics: Principles and Practice* (Philadelphia: W.B. Saunders & Company, 1961), 19. On the importance of this text, see Peter S. Vig, Review of Thomas Graber and Brainerd F. Swain, *Orthodontics: Current Principles and Techniques,* in *American Journal of Orthodontics* 87, no. 4 (April 1985): 347–8.

17 C. Fred Bodsworth, "Teeth Take a Detour," *Maclean's*, 15 Jan. 1948, 21, 40.

18 William Greaves, dir., *Putting It Straight: A Story of Crooked Teeth* (National Film Board, 1957).

19 R.O. Fisk, "Physiological and Socio-psychological Significance of Malocclusion," *JCDA* 29, no. 10 (Oct. 1963): 638.

20 J.F. Hickman, "An Orthodontic Priority Index Survey of 12-year-old Children in Forest Hill Village," submitted in partial fulfilment of the requirements for the Diploma Course in Orthodontics, University of Toronto, 1976, 38.

21 Allan Anderson, "Handsome Is as Orthodontist Does," *JCDA* 16, no. 7 (July 1950): 362.

22 "There Are No SAD Faces in This Dental Clinic," *Toronto Star*, 10 Feb. 1962, 47.

23 Joan Jacobs Brumberg, *Body Project: An Intimate History of American Girls* (New York: Vintage Books, 1997); Naomi Wolf, *The Beauty Myth: How Images of Beauty Are Used against Women* (New York: William Morrow & Co, 1991).

24 Marianne LaFrance and Marvin A. Hecht, "Gender and Smiling: A Metanalysis," in Agneta H. Fischer, ed., *Gender and Emotion: Social Psychological Perspectives* (Cambridge: Cambridge University Press, 2000), 118–42.

25 S. Robert Rutzen, "The Social Importance of Orthodontic Rehabilitation: Report of a Five Year Follow-up Study," *Journal of Health and Social Behavior* 14 (1973): 233–40; Rodney J. Klima, Joseph K. Wittemann, and James E. McIver, "Body Image, Self-Concept and the Orthodontic Patient," *American Journal of Orthodontics* 97, no. 5 (1979): 507–16; W.C. Shaw, M. Addy, and C. Ray, "Dental and Social Effects of Malocclusion and Effectiveness of Orthodontic Treatment: A Review," *Community Dental Oral Epidemiology* 8, no. 1 (1980): 36–45.

26 William R. Profitt, *Contemporary Orthodontics* (St Louis, MO: C.V. Mosby, 1986), 8–11.

27 Stephen F. Roth, Gideon Heo, Connie Varnhagen, Kenneth E. Glover, and Paul W. Major, "Job Satisfaction among Canadian Orthodontists," *American Journal of Orthodontics and Dentofacial Orthopedics* 123, no. 6 (2003): 695–700.

28 P.A. Konchak and R.E. McDermott, "Orthodontic Education and Practice in Canada: Perceptions of the Profession as Shown in a Recent Survey," *JCDA* 56, no. 6 (June 1990): 537–9.

29 "Marcine Can Live with Her Smile, but Can She Live with Her Teeth?," *Chatelaine*, Oct. 1981, 55.

30 "They're Showing You a Potentially Serious Health Problem," *Chatelaine*, Oct. 1983, 141.

31 Robin Harvey, "Ouch! Reality Bites," *Toronto Star*, 18 Nov. 1995, G1.

32 Ibid., G4.

33 Ibid., WS2.

34 Dave Truscott, "Brace Yourself," *Calgary Herald*, 1 Aug. 1981, B15.

35 Malcolm Yasny, "More Adults Wearing Braces," *Toronto Star*, 15 Nov. 1986, F4.

36 Leslie Scrivener, "More Adults Grinning and Baring a 'Metal' Smile," *Toronto Star*, 1 Aug. 1981, F2.

37 "Près de 40 p. de la clientèle des orthodontistes se compose maintenant d'adultes," *La Presse*, 12 Oct. 1991, K4.

38 Yasny, "More Adults Wearing Braces," F4.

39 Canada, Department of National Health and Welfare, *Dental Report: A Report from Nutrition Canada* (Ottawa, 1977).

40 Raina Telgemeier, *Smile* (New York: Scholastic, 2010). For biographical details, see Go Raina!, http://goraina.com/about/ <13 Sept. 2017>.

41 "'Backward' Teeth Braces Can't Be Seen," *Toronto Star*, 28 March 1982, H8.

42 Marlene Habib, "Looks-conscious Youngsters Embrace Braces," *Nanaimo Daily News*, 26 Oct. 2002, D5; Daniel Feist, "Beautiful Braces: A Mouth Full of Metal Has Become a New Status Symbol," *Montreal Gazette*, 26 Jan. 1998, E1.

43 Stephanie Nolen, "Brace Wearers Grin and Bare Colours," *Globe and Mail*, 2 Aug. 1993, A3.

44 Louis Malcmacher, "Invisalign," *Dental Economics* 95, no. 3 (March 2005): 65.

45 Laura Pratt, "Personal Affairs: Plenty of Reasons to Smile," *Globe and Mail*, 26 Aug. 1995, B20.

46 Kristin Rushowy, "Laser Technology Brightens up Smiles," *Toronto Star*, 13 Aug. 1998, 1.

47 Cheryl Cornacchia, "Whiten Your Teeth," *Kimberly Bulletin*, 3 March 2003, 11.

48 For example, in 2006 there were eight advertisements for oral-health-care products. One, for Arm and Hammer baking powder, promised to make teeth three shades whiter. Another was for Crest Vivid White Night Toothpaste, four were for Crest Whitestrips, and the last was for Listerine: "Nothing makes you feel more beautiful than your smile."

49 Karen von Hahn, "Noticed: Power Smiles," *Globe and Mail*, 6 July 2002, L3.
50 Susan Goldberg, "Thou Shalt Covet a Perfect Smile," *National Post*, 24 May 2003, SR6.
51 Christopher Mutter, "Blinded by the White: Remember When Pearly Whites Were the Colour of Pale Corn," *Edmonton Journal*, 12 July 2008, H3.
52 Åke Blomqvist and Frances Woolley, *Filling the Cavities: Improving the Efficacy and Equity of Canada's Dental Care System, Commentary No. 510, May 2018* (Toronto: C.D. Howe Institute, 2018), https://www.cdhowe.org/sites/default/files/attachments/research_papers/mixed/Final%20April%2026%20Commentary%20510.pdf <5 Sept. 2021>.
53 Eileen Travers, "Suddenly, Dentists Are Hip," *Montreal Gazette*, 19 Feb. 2005, G2.
54 Charles Pincus, "Appendix C: The Development of Dental Esthetics in the Motion Picture Industry," in Ronald Goldstein, ed., *Esthetics in Dentistry* (Philadelphia: Lippincott, 1976), 456–7.
55 Ronald Goldstein, *Change Your Smile* (Chicago: Quintessence Publishing, 1984), 36.
56 "Consumer Guide to Dentistry," https://www.yourdentistryguide.com/veneer-materials/ <5 Sept. 2021>.
57 Goldstein, *Change Your Smile*, 149.
58 For a list of problems and potential procedures, see Kenneth Aschheim and Barry G. Dale, *Esthetic Dentistry: A Clinical Approach to Techniques and Materials* (St Louis, MO: Mosby, 2001), 3–19.
59 Jan Ravensbergen, "Dental Procedures Will Brighten Smile for Some," *Montreal Gazette*, 5 March 1986, C2.
60 Iris Winston, "Cosmetic Dentistry Can Be a Life Changer," *Saskatoon Star Phoenix*, 14 April 2009, C2.
61 Iris Winston, "Cosmetic Dentistry Can Go beyond the Surface," *Montreal Gazette*, 14 April 2009, D10.
62 "Dentists Turn to Rebuilding Your Smile," *Ottawa Citizen*, 13 March 1987, A16.
63 Carola Vyhnak, "Look Who's Smiling Now," *Toronto Star*, 11 March 1993, FA6.
64 Jos V.M. Welie, "Do You Have a Healthy Smile? Ugliness as a Medical Indication for Dental and Surgical Cosmetic Treatment," *Medicine, Health Care and Philosophy* 2 (1999): 169–80.
65 "Toronto Academy of Cosmetic Dentistry," *Oral Health*, Aug. 1995, 16.
66 Travers, "Suddenly, Dentists Are Hip," G2.
67 "In Need of Last-Minute Dental Health Month Ideas?," *JCDA* 54, no. 3 (March 1988), 155; "Dental Awareness Program Update," *JCDA* 52, no. 3 (March 1986), 180; "Dental Awareness," *Globe and Mail*, 27 March 1985, B6.
68 Frank Faunce, "Esthetic Dentistry: A New Direction," *JCDA* 54, no. 4 (April 1988), 248.
69 Imtiaz Manji, "Dentistry: 'What, a Future?' or 'What a Future!'" *JCDA* 60, no. 10 (Nov. 1994), 863–5.

70 "Continuing Education Dental Seminars" advertisement. *Oral* Health 73, no. 1 (Jan, 1983), 52. This includes Cosmetic Dentistry through Bonding Seminar with "Drs. K. William Mopper and Norman Feigenbaum, two of the foremost authorities in the United States on bonding techniques and materials"; "Millennium Institute: In the course of just 6 days, 12 visionary dentists will make a beautiful transformation," *JCDA* 65, no. 1 (Jan. 1999): 62. "Invisalign" ad for courses, *Oral Health* 97, no. 1 (Jan. 2007), 40.

71 Art Chamberlain, "Cosmetic Dentistry Takes on a New Polish," *Toronto Star*, 26 Jan. 1994, A1.

72 Pierre Vallée, "Ils sont 162 "nouveaux" à s'incrire chaque année," *Le Devoir*, 12 Sept. 2004, H2.

73 Valeria V. Gordon, Amer Abu-Hanna, and Ivar A. Mjor, "Esthetic Dentistry in North American Dental Schools," *JCDA* 70, no. 4 (2004): 230a–230d.

74 "Dentists Turn to Rebuilding Your Smile," A16.

75 Irene Seiberling, "Smile Makeovers Growing in Popularity," *Regina Leader Post*, 15 May 2004, A10; Bonnie Bryan, "Local Dentist to Attend Cosmetic Dentistry Conference," *Cranbrook Townsman*, 26 April 2004, 3; Erik White, "The Quest for the Perfect Smile," *St. Catharines Standard*, 30 April 2005, A1.

76 Thomas Claridge, "Court Strikes down Regulations on Advertising by Dentists," *Globe and Mail*, 20 April 1988, A15; Kirk Martin, "Judge Rejects Strict Rules on Ads by Professionals," *Globe and Mail*, 22 June 1990, A1–A2.

77 Kirk Martin, "Dentists' Regulations Called Violation of Free Expression," *Globe and Mail*, 22 June 1990, A1. The Supreme Court ruling appears at [1990] 2 SCR 232.

78 In 1991–92, approximately one-quarter of all ads mentioned cosmetic services. By 2000, well over half of all advertising dentists indicated that they did cosmetic work. *Toronto Yellow Pages Household* (2000), 392–411; *Toronto Yellow Pages Household* (1991), 359–75.

79 The Don Valley Dental Centre advertised "Whitening, Veneers, Bridges, Crowns, Dentures, Implants and Gum Therapy" and featured three smiling couples of various ages and two children. Altima Dental Care highlighted its "Beautiful Smiles," while Yonge Eglinton Dental said that "We care for your smile" and featured a smiling couple, a smiling woman, and mother and son. *Yellow Pages (Toronto Central East) Household* (2005), 387–9.

80 David T. Ozar and David J. Sokol, *Dental Ethics at Chairside: Professional Principles and Practical Applications* (Washington, DC: Georgetown University Press, 2007), 282.

81 Ray E. McDermott, "Demand and Supply of Dental Services," *JCDA* 52, no. 12 (Dec. 1986): 994.

82 D.W. Lewis, "Dental Manpower Supply and Demand Projections and Changing Demography and Dental Disease," *JCDA* 52, no. 1 (Jan. 1986): 34.

83 Canada, *Health Personnel in Canada 1992* (Ottawa: Health Information

Division, Policy and Consultation Division, Minister of Supply and Services Canada, 1995), 48.

84 Canada, *Canada Health Manpower Inventory* (Ottawa: National Health and Welfare, 1980), 40.

85 Jan Wong, "Fluoride Has Dentists Frowning," *Globe and Mail*, 21 March 1996, A1.

86 Ibid.

87 Oskar Sykora, *Maritime Dental College and Dalhousie Faculty of Dentistry: A History* (Bedford: Nova Scotia Dental Association, 1991), 139–40.

88 Paul Wells, "Dental School Supported," *Montreal Gazette*, 3 Aug. 1991, 3; Kate Dunn, "McGill to Close Its Dentistry School," *Montreal Gazette*, 18 July 1991, 3; Kate Dunn, "Plan to Close Dental School Generates a Windfall," *Montreal Gazette*, 16 Oct. 1992, A1.

89 Jeff Lee, "New UBC President 'A Star,'" *Vancouver Sun*, 20 Nov. 1996, A4.

90 Maureen Marud, "Dental Patients Asked to Join Fight to Save College," *Saskatoon Star-Phoenix*, 2 March 1991, 3; David Yanko, "Dentistry College's Uncertain Future Prompts One of Two Senior Vacancies," *Saskatoon Star-Phoenix*, 8 Jan.1992, 2.

91 "Tuition," University Archives and Special Collections, University of Saskatchewan, https://library.usask.ca/archives/campus-history/tuition.php <5 Sept. 2021>.

92 "Tuition Fee Rise at Varsity Ranges from $29 to $70," *Globe and Mail*, 22 May 1951, 1.

93 "A Dental Investment," *Globe and Mail*, 5 March 1971, 3.

94 Caroline Alphonso, "U of T Approves Fee Hike of up to 5 per cent," *Globe and Mail*, 12 May 2000, A20.

95 Ken Neuman, "Cosmetic Imaging: A Look into the Future – Now!," *JCDA* 54, no. 4 (April 1988), 259. A later article also urged dentists to place a copy in the patients' waiting area. David S. Philip, "Incorporating Cosmetic Dentistry into a General Practice," *JCDA* 60, no. 8 (Aug. 1994), 682.

96 Imtiaz Mani, "Who's Minding the Store?," *JCDA* 62, no. 5 (May 1996), 409–10. A similar article is Murray Chantler, "The 'Not Busy' Syndrome," *Oral Health* 80, no. 8 (1990), 3.

97 *Sixty Minutes*, https://www.youtube.com/watch?v=rF_y4KlUB-k <5 Sept. 2021>.

98 Mark Lowey, "Dentists 'Stifling Debate, Analysis,'" *Calgary Herald*, 19 July 1992, A3.

99 Murray Vimy, *Your Toxic Teeth* (Calgary: Murray Vimy, 2000), first pub. 1993.

100 Steven Judd Sadowsky, "An Overview of Treatment Considerations for Esthetic Restorations: A Review of the Literature," *Journal of Prosthetic Dentistry* 96, no. 6 (Dec. 2006): 433–42. For articles on people having amalgam fillings removed, see Katherine Dedyna, "Heave Ho, Silver," *Victoria Times-Colonist*, 21 March 2003, B6.

101 Ronald Goldstein, *Esthetics in Dentistry*, 2nd ed. (Hamilton, ON, and London: B.C. Decker Inc, 1998), 10–11.

102 Howard E. Strassler, "Insights and Innovations: Esthetic Diagnosis," *Journal of Esthetic and Restorative Dentistry* 4, no. 2 (March 1992): 64–6; J. Dzierzak, "Achieving the Optimal Perio-esthetic Result: The Team Approach," *Journal of the American Dental Association* 123, no. 5 (May 1992): 41–8.

103 Goldstein, *Esthetics in Dentistry*, 2nd ed., 18.

104 Ibid., 52.

105 Ibid., 51–8.

106 Carlos Quiñonez, Rafael Figueiredo, Amir Azarpazhoo, and David Locker, "Public Preferences for Seeking Publicly Financed Dental Care and Professional Preferences for Structuring It," *Community Dentistry and Oral Epidemiology* 38, no. 2 (2010): 152–8. Such observations are not new. In 1972, at a weekly clinic in Saskatoon, a dentist and two dental students provided "transients" with dental care. They noted: "Whilst this venture has started only recently it has shown that transients are often too ashamed to attend a regular dental office even when they have the money." "Extramural Clinics," *Dalhousie Dental Journal* (1972): 11.

107 Ian Howarth, "Spa Dentistry Keeps Patient's Comfort in Mind," *Montreal Gazette*, 29 April 2009, D7.

108 Wong, "Fluoride Has Dentists Frowning," A1.

109 David Graham, "Although the Fashion Industry Has Consistently Promoted the Chic Factor of Pouting and Sulking, a New Cheerier Mood Is Invading," *Canadian Press*, 30 Nov. 2000, n.p.

110 Lilianne Lacroix, "Quand le cabinet du dentiste devient un spa," *La Presse*, 25 May 2003, B2.

111 Brian Morton, "Dental Salon Works on Entire Face," *Vancouver Sun*, 7 April 2008, C7.

112 Kathy Davis, *Reshaping the Female Body: The Dilemma of Cosmetic Surgery* (New York: Routledge, 1995), 18–19.

113 Canadian Medical Association, *Plastic Surgery Profile* (Ottawa: CMA, 2018), https://www.cma.ca/sites/default/files/2019-01/plastic-surgery-e.pdf <5 Sept. 2021>.

114 Lianne George, "Presto Chango," *Maclean's*, 26 April 2004, 40.

115 Michael Schneider, "Fox Sees True Ratings Beauty in 'The Swan,'" *Variety*, 29 April 2004, https://variety.com/2004/scene/markets-festivals/fox-sees-true-ratings-beauty-in-the-swan-1117904047/ <5 Sept. 2021>.

116 For the class dynamics of *Extreme Makeover*, see Cressida J. Heyes, "Cosmetic Surgery and the Television Makeover," *Feminist Media Studies* 7, no. 1 (2007): 17–32.

117 Tom Hedge, "Dentistry and the Extreme Makeover," *Dental Economics*, 1 Sept. 2003, https://www.dentaleconomics.com/science-tech/oral-medicine-

anesthetics-and-the-oral-systemic-connection/article/16387572/dentistry-and-the-extreme-makeover <5 Sept. 2021>.

118 Barry Polansky, *The Complete Dentist: Positive Leadership and Communication Skills for Success* (Newark, NJ: Wiley-Blackwell, 2017), 50.

119 Alexander C.L. Holden, Barry Gibson, and Heiko Spallek, "Embarrassing Realities: The Portrayal of Reality TV 'Dentertainment,'" *Community Dental Health* 36 (2018): 46–54.

120 This episode did emphasize brushing teeth and cutting down on sugar. "Extreme Makeover: Dr. Bill Dorfman Repairs Extreme Tooth Decay," https://www.youtube.com/watch?v=n1aIuTUOmT8 <5 Sept. 2021>. It also showed the makeover recipient how to brush and floss. See another clip here: https://www.youtube.com/watch?v=uusrdP9D1yg <5 Sept. 2021>.

121 Gordon J. Christensen, "The Perception of Professionalism in Dentistry: Further Reflections on a Lively Topic," *Journal of the American Dental Association* 133 (April 2002): 499–501.

122 Richard J. Simonsen, "Commerce versus Care: Troubling Trends in the Ethics of Esthetic Dentistry," *Dental Clinics of North America* 51 (2007): 281–7.

123 I. Ahmad, "Risk Management in Clinical Practice. Part 5. Ethical Considerations for Dental Enhancement Procedures," *British Dental Journal* 209 (2010): 207–14.

124 Donald F. Mulcahy, "Cosmetic Dentistry: Is It Really Health Care?," *JCDA* 66, no. 2 (Feb. 2000): 86–7.

125 Arthur Schafer, "Danger in Drilling for Gold Teeth," *Globe and Mail*, 25 July 1991, A15.

126 Welie, "Do You Have a Healthy Smile?," 169–80.

127 Ahmad, "Risk Management in Clinical Practice. Part 5," 207–14.

128 Interview with D.B., 9 Sept. 2013; Brian Saby, "The Art of Dentistry," *Red Deer Advocate*, 21 Nov. 2001, 19; Daisy Goldstein, "Art with Teeth," *Montreal Gazette*, 12 Jan. 2006, 47.

129 Stephen Hancocks, "The Ethics of Cosmetics," *British Dental Journal* 211, no. 11 (10 Dec. 2011): 501.

130 Ken Glick, "Cosmetic Dentistry Is Still Dentistry," *JCDA* 66, no. 2 (Feb. 2000): 88.

131 Alexander C.L. Holden, "Cosmetic Dentistry: A Socioethical Evaluation," *Bioethics* 32 (2018): 606.

132 "The Changing Face of Oral Health," *Globe and Mail*, 2 April 2007, CDA1.

Conclusion

1 Canadian Dental Association, *The State of Orsl Health in Canada* (Ottawa: Canadian Dental Association, 2017).

2 Minn Y. Yoon, Carla Ickert, Susan E. Slaughter, Christina Lengyel, Natalie Carrier, and Heather Keller, "Oral Health Status of Long-term Care Residents

in Canada: Results of a National Cross-sectional Study," *Gerodontology* 35 (2018): 359–64.

3 Canadian Dental Association, *The State of Oral Health*.

4 Canadian Centre for Policy Alternatives, *Putting Money Where Our Mouth Is: The Future of Dental Care in Canada* (Ottawa: Canadian Centre for Policy Alternatives, 2011).

5 "Access to Care Initiatives by Provincial Dental Associations," https://www.cda-adc.ca/stateoforalhealth/pdaaccess/ <10 Sept. 2021>.

6 Carlos Quiñonez et al., *An Environmental Scan of Publicly Financed Dental Care in Canada* (Toronto: Community Dental Health Services Research Unit, 2015), 15.

7 Paul Hunter, "A Decade Later, He's Still Smiling," *Toronto Star*, 30 Oct. 2017, A3; "Healthy Smiles Ontario Program," https://www.toronto.ca/311/knowledgebase/kb/docs/articles/public-health/dental-and-oral-health-services/healthy-smiles-ontario-program.html#:~:text=On%20October%201%2C%20 2010%20the,eligible%20children%2017%20and%20under <10 Sept. 2021>.

8 Parliamentary Budget Office, Cost Estimate of a Federal Dental Care Program for Uninsured Canadians (Parliamentary Budget Office, 2020), https://www.pbo-dpb.gc.ca/web/default/files/Documents/Reports/RP-2021-028-M/RP-2021-028-M_en.pdf <21 Jan. 2021>.

9 Brandon Doucet, "Dental Care in Canada More Closely Resembles a Private U.S.-style Healthcare System Than One Worthy of Applause," *Passage*, 13 Oct. 2020, https://readpassage.com/as-a-dentist-i-know-canada-needs-universal-public-dental-care/ <10 Sept. 2021>.

10 "Singh Renews Pledge of Federal Dental Care, Says Liberals Take Atlantic Canada for Granted," 4 Sept. 2021, https://www.cbc.ca/news/politics/singh-dental-care-1.6165041 <23 Sept. 2021>.

11 Carlos Quiñonez, David Locker, Laurel Sherret, Paul Grootendorst, Amir Azarpazhooh, and Rafael Figueiredo, *An Environmental Scan of Publicly Financed Dental Care in Canada* (Toronto: Community Dental Health Services Research Unit, 2015), https://www.caphd.ca/sites/default/files/FINAL%20-%202015%20Environmental%20Scan%20-%20ENGLISH%20-%2016%20Feb%2016.pdf <5 July 2021>.

12 Carlos Quiñonez, *The Politics of Dental Care in Canada* (Toronto: Canadian Scholars Press, 2021), 256–343.

13 L. McLaren, S. Patterson, S. Thawer, P. Faris, C. McNeil, M.L. Potestio, and L. Shwart, "Exploring the Short-term Impact of Community Water Fluoridation Cessation on Children's Dental Caries: A Natural Experiment in Alberta, Canada," *Public Health* 146 (May 2017): 56–64; "Cavity Rates Rising in Windsor, Say Health Officials," CBC News, 21 April 2016, https://www.cbc.ca/news/canada/windsor/windsor-tooth-decay-fluoride-1.3546919 <10 Sept. 2021>; "Coming Clean: Good Hygiene Key to Curbing Rising Tooth Decay Rates in Kids," *National Post*, 10 April 2012, https://nationalpost.com/health/

coming-clean-good-hygiene-key-to-curbing-rising-tooth-decay-rates-in-kids <10 Sept. 2021>.

14 Emily Wong, *The Real Cost of Removing Water Fluoridation* (Toronto: Wellesley Institute, 2013).

15 "How Publicly Financed Dental Care Is Delivered in Canada vs. the United States," Webinar by Coalition for Dentalcare, 17 Nov. 2020.

16 Joanne N. Walton et al., "The Burden of Debt for Canadian Dental Students: Part 4," *JCDA* 72, no. 10 (Dec.–Jan. 2007): 913a–913e.

Index